The Source®
for Children's Voice Disorders

by Nancy B. Swigert

Skill	Ages	Grades
▪ voice	▪ 5 through 14	▪ K through 9

Evidence-Based Practice

- ASHA (2005) supports voice therapy for treatment of dysphonia. Voice therapy is a preferred behavioral intervention before pursing invasive medical interventions, such as vocal fold injections or surgery. Voice therapy can improve surgical outcomes with certain types of etiologies, such as vocal fold nodules.

- Ramig and Verdolini (1998) found evidence to support voice therapy for voice disorders of various etiologies. Speech-language pathologists (SLPs) have the educational training and clinical experience to assist an individual with a voice disorder improve his/her voice, leading to improved functional communication, social interactions, willingness to participate in school, and psychological well-being.

- Effective voice therapy for children needs to involve multiple components, including education on how the voice functions, etiology, contributing behaviors, vocal hygiene, and direct voice therapy. A multidisciplinary team approach, including parents, teachers, and medical professionals, will produce the most comprehensive results (Hooper, 2004).

- Use of instrumentation and verbal feedback from the SLP is highly desirable for a child to learn correct and incorrect use of voice production (Harvey, 1996).

- Paradoxical vocal fold motion is often diagnosed in children and adolescent athletes who are labeled "high achievers." The SLP can play an important role in education and intervention for this complex and often misdiagnosed disorder (Mathers-Schmidt, 2001).

The Source for Children's Voice Disorders incorporates these principles and is also based on expert professional practice.

References

American Speech-Language-Hearing Association. (ASHA). (2005). *The use of voice therapy in the treatment of dysphonia* [Technical Report]. Retrieved August 4, 2009, from www.asha.org/policy

Harvey, G.L. (1996). Treatment of voice disorders in medically complex children. *Language, Speech, and Hearing Services in Schools, 27,* 282-291.

Hooper, C.R. (2004). Treatment of voice disorders in children. *Language, Speech, and Hearing Services in Schools, 35,* 320-326.

Mathers-Schmidt, B.A. (2001). Paradoxical vocal fold motion: A tutorial on a complex disorder and the speech-language pathologist's role. *American Journal of Speech-Language Pathology, 10,* 111-125.

Ramig, L.O., & Verdolini, K. (1998). Treatment efficacy: Voice disorders. *Journal of Speech, Language, and Hearing Research, 41,* S101-S116.

LinguiSystems®

LinguiSystems, Inc.
3100 4th Avenue
East Moline, IL 61244
800-776-4332

FAX: 800-577-4555
Email: service@linguisystems.com
Web: linguisystems.com

Printed in the U.S.A.

ISBN 10: 0-7606-0617-X
ISBN 13: 978-0-7606-0617-9

About the Author

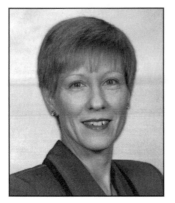

Nancy B. Swigert, M.A., CCC-SLP, is president of Swigert & Associates, Inc., a private practice that has been providing services in the Lexington, Kentucky area for over 25 years. She evaluates and treats children and adults with voice disorders through her company's contractual agreement with Central Baptist Hospital. She works closely with several otolaryngology practices as well as a pulmonary group. Nancy is the author of five other products for LinguiSystems, *The Source for Dysphagia*, *The Source for Dysarthria*, *The Source for Pediatric Dysphagia*, *The Source for Reading Fluency*, and *The Early Intervention Kit*. She is very active in the American Speech-Language-Hearing Association, including serving as its president in 1998 and president of the American Speech-Language-Hearing Foundation in 2004-2005.

Dedication

This book is dedicated to my mother, June Ballman, and my brother, Randy Ballman. Long before I even knew what a speech-language pathologist was, or that I wanted to be one, Randy provided my first exposure to voice disorders in children when he screamed so much as an infant that he developed vocal nodules. His nodules were surgically removed, perhaps because at that time there weren't speech-language pathologists easily accessible in schools or in clinics. I'm happy to report that he has a healthy voice now. Surely my mom deserves recognition for putting up with that much screaming . . . and for nurturing the two of us over the years.

A special thank-you also goes to my husband, Keith, who became a second nurturer to me 30 years ago this year.

Acknowledgments

Geri Cadle, executive assistant extraordinaire, for helping to keep me on track with researching and writing this book

Melinda Spurlock, for double and triple checking references and hunting down articles

Lonnie Wright and the staff at the Central Baptist Hospital Medical Library for the uncanny ability to find needed references in a flash

Edited by Lauri Whiskeyman
Layout by Jamie Bellagamba
Illustrations by Margaret Warner
Cover Design by Jason Platt

Table of Contents

Table of Contents, *continued*

Table of Contents, continued

Introduction

Voice disorders in children probably occur more frequently than voice disorders in adults. Estimates of the prevalence of voice disorders in school-age children range from 6% (Hull et al. 1976) to a high of 23% (Silverman & Zimmer 1975). Despite this high prevalence, many speech-language pathologists (SLPs) working primarily with children rarely see a child with a voice disorder. Wilson (1979) noted that although 6-9% of elementary school children have voice disorders, only 1% of children on SLPs caseloads have voice disorders. Andrews and Summers (2002) hypothesized that this may be related to the difficulty in getting the child examined by a physician before beginning therapy. It may also be related to an acceptance that the child "has always sounded that way." Sometimes parents and teachers are so accustomed to hearing the child's hoarse voice that it doesn't sound "abnormal" to them.

Whatever the reason, the fact that SLPs don't see lots of children with voice disorders may contribute to a lack of confidence in evaluating and treating these children. Yet it can be fun and rewarding to treat children with voice disorders — they generally demonstrate quick progress and get better. SLPs should have a critical role in the management of children with voice disorders. Often, behavioral voice treatment is the preferred treatment.

In all areas of practice, it is important that clinicians use an evidence-based approach to treatment. This means that we should carefully analyze evaluation and treatment techniques to determine if they have been shown to be efficacious. Voice disorders are no exception, and solid research studies do exist on treatment efficacy, though often not specific to the pediatric population. For example, Ramig and Verdolini (1998) wrote a review article on the efficacy of treatment for voice disorders. In this article, they indicated that the consensus is that "children with vocal hyperfunction and vocal nodules should receive voice treatment." In a study of 31 school children with vocal nodules, 84% (after six months) had reduced nodule size and 65% had normal larynges (Deal et al. 1976). Allen et al. (1991) also reported that voice treatment was effective in treating vocal nodules. Vocal hygiene programs have also been found to reduce the number of children perceived as hoarse (Nilson & Schneiderman 1983).

This book is not designed to teach you everything you need to know about voice disorders in children. There are many excellent, comprehensive textbooks that you may want to use to supplement the information provided here. This book is designed to serve as a reference tool and to give you techniques, methods, and materials (including a PowerPoint presentation on the accompanying CD that is designed to educate children about the voice) to use with children who have typical voice disorders. Unusual or low incidence voice problems (e.g., paralysis of vocal folds) are not addressed. This book should be useful to SLPs in school or healthcare settings who see children from kindergarten to middle school. Many of the techniques described can be used with older children, though the handouts may need to be adapted in some cases to be more age appropriate. In addition, this book does not deal with voice problems unique to adolescents (e.g., puberphonia).

Chapter 1 describes the kinds of things that can go wrong with the voice. You'll find descriptions of problems related to voice abuse/misuse and the consequences (e.g., vocal nodules) of such abuse. Medically-related causes of voice problems (e.g., upper respiratory infections, GERD) are also addressed, as well as congenital medical disorders with related voice problems (e.g., cleft palate, cerebral palsy).

Clinical evaluation of the voice (discussed in Chapter 2) is an important step in analyzing the perceptual characteristics of the child's voice. This analysis will provide valuable information for developing a treatment plan. Chapter 3 gives some basic information about instrumental evaluations of voice disorders. It does not provide enough information to prepare you to perform such instrumental evaluations. However, it should help you understand reports of instrumental evaluations you receive from others, and to determine when and why you might want to refer a child for a comprehensive instrumental evaluation.

The combined information from both types of evaluation forms the basis for treatment planning. Many other factors must be considered, however, when planning treatment (Chapter 4) for children. One of the challenges is motivating the child to change something he may not perceive as a problem. Behavior management techniques need to be utilized and other adults need to be enlisted in the effort to change the behaviors. The framework for using short-term goals and treatment objectives is also addressed in this chapter.

Most voice problems presented by children will be problems of hyperfunction, which Boone et al. (2005) described as "the involvement of excessive muscle force and physical effort in the systems of respiration, phonation, and resonance." A description of types of hyperfunction and the relationship of hyperfunction to the development of organic problems is described in Chapter 5. The fundamentals for treating hyperfunction are explained, along with several specific techniques.

Since many children with hyperfunctional voice disorders are abusing their voices, Chapter 6 provides detailed information about behavior management strategies that can be used to modify vocally abusive behaviors. The appendices in this chapter include forms that should help you in collecting data on these behaviors.

Chapters 7, 8, and 9 provide more in-depth information and treatment strategies about three specific physiologic functions that contribute to voice production: respiration, phonation, and oral-nasal resonance. You'll find yourself referring to these chapters for the child who has an isolated problem with these functions or for the child who needs extra practice in these areas to supplement treatment of a hyperfunctional voice pattern.

Chapter 10 describes Paradoxical Vocal Fold Dysfunction. This really isn't a voice disorder (though some children with PVFD may have an accompanying voice problem). However, it is a problem with the larynx, and a book on voice disorders seemed the logical place to include information on how to treat it.

I hope you find *The Source for Children's Voice Disorders* to be a helpful resource and a trigger to seek out more information about voice disorders in children.

Nancy

8

Disorders of Voice: What Can Go Wrong

Voice disorders in children may be related to a variety of etiologies. Understanding the causes of voice disorders will help you do a better job collecting case history information, determining a prognosis, and planning treatment.

There are different classification systems to organize the way we think about voice disorders. Aronson (1990) divided disorders into functional and organic. Boone et al. (2005) described the problem with a functional vs. organic division (one used by Boone in earlier editions), indicating the terms may be too broad to adequately describe voice problems. They revised their classification system to a three-way system: functional, neurological, and organic. Stemple et al. (2000) described common etiologic factors such as vocal misuse, medically-related etiologies, primary disorder etiologies, and personality-related etiologies. In this chapter, we'll describe disorders of voice in three ways:

1. Voice abuse/misuse (e.g., shouting, hyperfunctional use of the mechanism) and consequences of vocal abuse (e.g., vocal nodules)

2. Medically-related causes of voice problems (e.g., upper respiratory infections, gastroesophageal reflux disease [GERD])

3. Congenital medical disorders with related voice problems (e.g., cleft palate, cerebral palsy)

1. Disorders Related to Vocal Abuse and Misuse

Vocal abuse

Vocal abuse occurs when the vocal folds are forcibly brought together. Wilson (1979) distinguished between vocal abuse and misuse and defined *abuse* as sudden straining of the voice or chronic use of harmful voice practices. If this chronic, harmful use continues over time, physical changes to the vocal mechanism can result. These changes might include swelling, strain, thickening, and even growths on the vocal folds.

Children engage in many vocal behaviors that would be considered abusive. These include:

- shouting
- screaming
- talking too loudly
- making loud or tense noises (e.g., car sounds)
- coughing
- throat clearing

Coughing may be occurring because the child has a medical problem (e.g., upper respiratory infection, asthma, cold). It is also a symptom of GERD. If the cough is related to a medical problem, the child should be receiving treatment from a physician. However, sometimes a cough has become an habitual behavior after the

9

medical problem that initially provoked the cough has resolved. A child may also cough because he has a sensation of something in his throat. This sensation may be caused by a vocal pathology. For example, if the child has nodules or even just mucous in his throat, a cough might be his response to the sensation. If the cough is not something that can be remediated medically, it is appropriate to treat the cough as an abusive behavior that needs to be eliminated (Blager et al. 1988).

Just as cough may be related to a primary medical problem, throat clearing can also be a habit, and one that is very abusive to the voice. Children will often clear their throats in response to a sensation that something is in their throats. Throat clearing brings the vocal folds together very forcefully. It is one of the most common forms of vocal abuse (Wilson 1979).

Vocal misuse

Vocal misuse differs from abuse. *Misuse* can be described as abnormal patterns of use the child develops. Many of these patterns will be related to hyperfunctional use of the mechanism. Boone et al. (2005) described vocal hyperfunction as "the involvement of excessive muscle force and physical effort in the systems of respiration, phonation, and resonance" (p. 8). If that is the case, the abnormal patterns can also result in physical changes to the mechanism as described above. Although Wilson (1979) described misuse related to incorrect pitch and loudness, the misuse may occur in respiration, phonation, and/or resonance. Hyperfunction of the mechanism may be observed in respiratory muscles, phonatory muscles, and even in the oral cavity. (See Chapter 5, pages 70-82 for more information on hyperfunction.) Some of the problems described below are clearly hyperfunctional in nature.

Respiration Although most children with voice disorders are probably using normal respiration to support speech (Aronson 1990), some children may develop abnormal patterns. For example, the child may breathe with shallow breathing, characterized by excess movement in the clavicular region. The voice may sound breathy or low in intensity. A child might also speak on low air. That is, at the end of an utterance, instead of taking another breath, the child continues to speak. This behavior results in increased tension of the laryngeal muscles. Often children who are speaking on low air are also talking too fast, and are trying to get as much talking in as quickly as they can. When a child talks on low air, the respiratory system and the phonatory system may be used in a hyperfunctional way.

Phonation Some children may use a hard glottal attack, which is a quick and forceful closure of the vocal folds with explosive release of the air. This behavior results in increased tension of the mechanism. Other children may use breathy phonation, allowing air to escape before closing the vocal folds for phonation. Breathy phonation requires extra tension in the folds as well. Both hard glottal attack and breathy phonation may be forms of hyperfunction.

A child may also use a pitch that is too low (often described as glottal fry) or too high. Too high a pitch is accompanied by an elevated larynx caused by excess muscular tension. If the child is not using an habitual pitch in the optimum range, it may put undue stress on the vocal mechanism.

The child may also exhibit pitch breaks. Pitch breaks are most commonly seen in adolescents experiencing pubertal growth; however, voice disorders in adolescents are beyond the scope of this book. The other cause of pitch breaks is vocal hyperfunction with speech at an inappropriate pitch level. Boone et al. (2005) indicated that if the child is speaking too high in his frequency range, his voice may break down one octave. If the child is speaking at an inappropriately low frequency, his voice may break one octave higher.

> *Resonance* Most resonance problems are related to a physical problem (i.e., velopharyngeal incompetence), but some children may exhibit a hypernasal resonance out of habit rather than a faulty mechanism. If the child is losing air out the nasal cavity, he may increase tension in the larynx to compensate.
>
> Resonance related to voice disorders does not refer only to hypernasality, but also to the balance of oral and nasal resonance. The term *resonance* is also used to describe the impact that the entire vocal tract has on resonance of vocal quality. For example, a child who speaks through clenched muscles of the face with very little movement of the articulators will present with a voice that resonates differently than if the child uses good movement of the articulators with a relaxed jaw.

Most often the child will exhibit more than one of these misuse behaviors. It is the cumulative effect that may result in the voice disorder. Vocal misuse has been identified as the most common cause of voice disorders. Though his clients were not limited to children, Cooper (1973) found 36.6% of his clients had voice disorders associated with vocal misuse and Brodnitz (1971) cited 25.8% of his clients. Helping the child identify all the situations in which these behaviors occur is an integral part of the voice evaluation.

Physical changes to the vocal mechanism as a result of vocal abuse or misuse

Swelling (traumatic laryngitis)

Boone et al. (2005) described swelling of the vocal folds that can result from excessive, strained vocalizations. Swelling of the folds can occur after one occurrence of prolonged vocal abuse (e.g., yelling at a sporting event), and can also result from continuous irritation (e.g., allergies, vocal abuse). The edges of the vocal folds become swollen and irritated.

If the swelling is caused by one occurrence of vocal abuse, simply allowing the vocal folds to rest usually returns the voice to normal. This is one of the few occasions in which voice rest is appropriately prescribed. Children placed on voice rest to recover from traumatic laryngitis should not whisper because the whisper is a hyperfunctional behavior. The ventricular, or false folds, may even be brought into function during the whisper, indicating the extent of the hyperfunction (e.g., overdriving the vocal mechanism) (Pearl & McCall 1986).

Thickening

Thickening is a broad-based lesion that may cover the anterior two-thirds of the margins of the vocal folds. Boone et al. (2005) indicated that there are two types of vocal fold thickening:

- early tissue reaction (swelling) to trauma
- the result of prolonged irritation that results in degeneration of the vocal folds, known as *polypoid degeneration*

Andrews (1986) reported other causes of thickening (see section on Medically Related problems, pages 13-15).

Vocal nodules

Nodules are generally bilateral and are found on the glottal margin at the anterior and middle third junction. When nodules are first developing, they may be soft and pliable, but with continuous abuse and misuse, the nodules become larger and harder, sometimes described as callous-like. Vocal nodules are the most common benign lesion on the vocal folds (Boone et al. 2005).

The voice of a child with vocal nodules will sound hoarse but also somewhat breathy because air is escaping through the edges of the vocal folds when they approximate. Because the vocal nodules add mass to the folds, the voice may also sound somewhat lower in pitch. A child with nodules may clear his throat a lot because he has the sensation that something is in his throat. In preadolescents, nodules are more common in boys, most likely because boys tend to engage in noisier vocal behaviors than girls.

Whether the nodules are relatively new and soft, or more established, a course of voice therapy is typically indicated. Even if more advanced nodules need to be removed surgically, it is important for the child to undergo voice therapy. Otherwise, the child may resume the same vocal abuse and misuse after the surgery, causing the vocal nodules to return.

Vocal fold polyps

Polyps are rarely seen in children (Stemple et al. 2000). Polyps are more typically seen on one side than bilaterally, and can be caused by vocal hyperfunction. These lesions are usually soft and often fluid filled. Polyps may be caused by a one-time vocal abusive event, such as loud screaming. Two types of polyps are:

- sessile (broad-based)
- pedunculated (narrow-based)

The voice of the child with a polyp may be much worse than that of a child with a nodule because the polyp creates greater interference with vocal fold closure.

Polyps may be removed surgically, but the same caution applies that if the child does not change whatever vocal behaviors caused the polyps to begin with, the polyps may recur after surgery. Polyps can be eliminated with voice therapy instead of surgery (Boone et al. 2005).

Contact ulcers

Contact ulcers are found on the posterior one-third of the vocal folds where the arytenoid cartilages are located. Unlike nodules and polyps, contact ulcers are often associated with pain. Contact ulcers can be caused by very forceful closure of the arytenoid cartilages, usually associated with low-pitched phonation and a hard glottal attack (Boone et al. 2005). However, contact ulcers may also be caused by laryngo-pharyngeal reflux. The term *granuloma* may also be used to describe contact ulcers.

2. Disorders with Medically-Related Causes

Infectious laryngitis

The swelling associated with laryngitis was described on page 11. Typically laryngitis occurs with an upper respiratory infection or sinusitis. Laryngitis can have a viral or bacterial cause. Physicians will often prescribe voice rest and hydration for cases of infectious laryngitis along with medical treatment if the origin is bacterial. In children, laryngitis may be accompanied by narrowing of the subglottic airway. This causes a sharp cough, hoarseness, and inhalatory stridor (noisy sounds when breathing in called *croup*). An attack of croup can last 30 minutes to an hour and repeat attacks are common (Stemple et al. 2000).

Chronic respiratory illnesses

Chronic respiratory problems such as asthma or obstructive pulmonary disease can directly or indirectly contribute to voice disorders. The child may wheeze or cough. The coughing may cause hoarseness, but the hoarseness may also be caused by poor respiratory support or even by the medications given to treat the problem (Stemple et al. 2000). For example, inhaled corticosteroids may contribute to bowing of the vocal folds, which could result in higher habitual pitch and perceived hoarseness (Watkin & Ewanowski 1979).

Thickening of the vocal folds

Thickening of the vocal folds was also described on page 11. However, there can be medical causes for thickening of the vocal folds. Andrews (1986) indicated that chronic upper respiratory problems and endocrine imbalance are two possible causes.

Contact ulcers/granuloma

Contact ulcers associated with abuse and misuse were described on page 12. There are two other common causes for granuloma:

- intubation during surgery
- gastric reflux

When a child is intubated, the breathing tube is placed into the trachea between the vocal folds which can cause damage to the vocal folds. This type of granuloma may need to be removed surgically. Continuous exposure to gastric acid through reflux can also cause the formation of granuloma. *Laryngo-pharyngeal reflux* is the term used to indicate that the refluxed material has moved up through the upper esophageal sphincter and into the pharynx and larynx. The related term *GERD* (gastroesophageal reflux) refers to reflux that stays in the esophagus.

Congenital and acquired cysts

Cysts are fluid-filled growths with an unclear etiology. They can occur anywhere in the membranous portion of the true vocal folds, in the laryngeal ventricle, or in the false vocal folds. They are usually unilateral, but may be bilateral. Thickening may occur on the fold opposite the cyst. Cysts do not respond to voice therapy. Surgical removal is required (Stemple et al. 2000).

Laryngeal web

A web is a growth between the two vocal folds. The web can make it difficult for the child to breathe and will cause the phonation to sound abnormal, often with a high pitched sound. Some webs are present at birth and are called *congenital webs*. These are corrected with immediate surgery and are sometimes followed with a tracheostomy that is placed temporarily until there is no chance of recurrence of the web. Acquired laryngeal webs may be caused by severe laryngeal infections or can even be a result of bilateral surgery on the vocal folds (Boone et al. 2005). Acquired webs are also corrected surgically.

Papilloma

These wart-like growths can occur anywhere in the upper aerodigestive tract but are most common on the vocal folds. They are caused by the human papilloma virus (HPV) infection. Onset is usually in the first decade of life. There is a link between HPV in the child's mother during pregnancy and papilloma in children, though the link is not fully understood. Papilloma is a good example of why it is important to refer for medical evaluation of the larynx before treating any child with hoarseness. These growths can become malignant and there is the possibility of airway compromise. The growths are removed surgically when they interfere with the child's breathing, but may continue to recur. Voice therapy may help to reduce the severity and spread in children if the children also avoid hyperfunctional voice use (Bouchayer et al. 1985). Voice therapy may also be helpful after surgery to help the child recover optimal voice use (Stemple et al. 2000). Papilloma usually disappear during puberty.

Sulcus vocalis

A sulcus on the vocal fold(s) is a ridge or furrow along the length of the medial surface of the vocal fold. Stemple (2000) indicated the etiology is uncertain but may be due to impaired embryologic maturation. A sulcus may be overlooked without videostroboscopic examination. Vocal quality may be mildly to severely impaired, depending on the stiffness of the vocal folds. Voice therapy may be of some help and surgery has had mixed results (Ringel & Chodzko-Zaijko 1987).

Paralysis

Paralysis of the vocal folds is a relatively common occurrence in children (Holinger & Brown 1967), representing 10% of all congenital anomalies of the larynx. It is caused by injury to the nerves that supply the vocal folds, most commonly central nervous system abnormalities, congenital cardiovascular disease, or unexplained local trauma (Rosin et al. 1990). Paralysis can be unilateral (usually due to trauma that can occur during surgery for cardiac abnormalities) or bilateral (usually neurological deficits) and the folds can be paralyzed in an abducted or adducted position. Some type of surgical procedure is often needed to correct the paralysis if function does not return spontaneously. If the vocal folds are paralyzed in an abducted position, it is likely that the voice will sound breathy. The child may compensate for this lack of closure by using a hyperfunctional voice which will cause the voice to sound hoarse/harsh. (See Chapter 5, pages 70-82 for more information on hyperfunction.)

Hyperfunction in reaction to the medically-related problem

When a child has an organic problem with his vocal folds, he may try to compensate for a less than ideal voice by pushing too hard (i.e., using excessive muscular tension) when talking. That is, he may develop a hyperfunctional voice pattern in reaction to the primary problem he has with the vocal folds and voice.

3. Voice Problems Caused by Congenital Medical Disorders

Cerebral palsy

Depending on the type of cerebral palsy, children may have distinctive voice characteristics. Some typical characteristics include forced or intermittent phonation, phonation on inhalation, difficulty coordinating phonation with respiration, impaired pitch control, breathiness, and some spasms of the vocal folds. Typically, hyperfunction of the vocal mechanism is noted with children who have spastic cerebral palsy and hypotension with children with athetoid cerebral palsy (Mysak 1980).

Cleft palate

Children with cleft palate (and with velopharyngeal insufficiency due to other causes) obviously have resonance problems, with hypernasality and nasal emission common. Their voices may be characterized by breathiness and reduced loudness. Aronson (1990) hypothesizes that the breathiness may be due to the child attempting to compensate for air that is lost out the nose by increasing airflow through the glottis. Some children may also develop hyperfunctional voice patterns as they overdrive the vocal folds and try to produce a louder voice. McWilliams et al. (1969) found a high incidence of vocal nodules in children with cleft palate.

Deafness

Children who are prelinguistically deaf often have an easily recognized vocal quality. This has been described as a cul-de-sac resonance. Other vocal characteristics associated with deafness and hearing impairment include pitch distortions and difficulty controlling loudness and rate.

Down Syndrome

Children with Down Syndrome have reduced muscle tone in all their muscles. Not surprisingly, then, their vocal quality is often breathy and rough and they present with hypernasal resonance (Montague & Hollien 1973).

Summary

Becoming familiar with different causes of voice disorders in children will help you in many ways. You will be better able to discuss the cause of the voice problem with the child and his family, be better prepared for discussions with otolaryngologists, and plan more effective intervention.

Clinical Evaluation of Voice

Multiple factors must be considered when analyzing the child's voice disorder. These factors include many things beyond the acoustic and perceptual information about the child's voice. Assessing the acoustic and perceptual information may or may not involve the use of sophisticated instrumentation. Because many speech-language pathologists (SLPs) who evaluate and treat children with voice disorders do not have access to such sophisticated instrumentation, that information has been included in a separate chapter (Chapter 3, pages 35-41). Even if you are not the clinician performing the instrumental assessment, it is important that you understand the type of information that can be obtained through the use of instrumental techniques. In this chapter, however, we focus on the clinical (i.e., non-instrumental) assessment.

Screening and Referrals

Screening

If you work in a preschool or school setting, you may identify students with voice disorders through screenings or you may receive referrals. If you routinely screen children for speech and language problems, it is easy to add a component to screen for voice disorders. While administering items to assess articulation and language skills, listen to the quality of the student's voice. Note the following about the student's voice:

- Is it harsh?
- Is it hoarse?
- Is it breathy?
- Is it too high or too low in pitch compared to peers?
- Does the student use an abnormally loud volume?
- Does the child strain to talk?
- Does the child have bad vocal habits (e.g., constant throat clearing, screaming)?

The s/z ratio can also be used as a screening of quality. Eckel and Boone (1981) found elevated s/z ratios greater than 1.4 in 95% of their patients with glottal margin pathologies (e.g., nodules, polyps). However, this is a "crude, quick appraisal technique" based on air wastage that would occur when the glottal margins don't meet (Boone et al. 2005). See a description of this technique on page 23.

Because voice problems may be transitory (e.g., the child's voice sounds hoarse one day because he didn't take his allergy medication and is fine the next), it is a good idea to re-screen the voice within a few weeks. During this time, you can gather information from the child's teacher concerning vocal habits. You could also send a form home to the parents to collect more information. *Observation of Child's Voice Use* (Appendix 2A, page 25) could be used to collect this information that will help you determine how to proceed. (See Chapter 4 for more information on how to utilize evaluation information to plan intervention). Develop a simple methodology for tracking students who need to be re-screened, such as listing the student's name on your calendar on the date you want to re-screen.

Referrals in school settings

In many school settings, SLPs do not screen children. They evaluate children when referred by the child's teacher. Teachers are familiar with the work SLPs do with children who have articulation, fluency, and language disorders. They may not be as familiar with what can be done for children with voice disorders. In addition, teachers may not be attuned to listening to the different features of a child's voice. For that reason, teachers may need some education about voice disorders in order to make appropriate referrals. As mentioned on page 16, *Observation of Child's Voice Use* (Appendix 2A, page 25) may also be helpful to teachers, coaches, and even parents in identifying voice problems in children. You might send the form home for the parents to provide information about their child's voice use away from the school setting. In addition, pages 169-172 and the CD accompanying this book contain a PowerPoint presentation designed to educate children about the voice. This presentation would be helpful to teachers as well.

Referrals in health care settings

In health care settings, the child is typically referred to the SLP by someone who has noted problems with the child's voice. This referral may come from a parent or from the child's primary care physician. In some instances, the child will have already been seen by an otolaryngologist, who makes the referral to the SLP.

Medical Evaluation

Any child with a voice disorder should be seen by a physician, "preferably in a discipline appropriate to the presenting complaint" (ASHA *Preferred Practice Patterns* 2004). Typically this means an otolaryngologist, but might mean a different specialist. For example, a pulmonologist might see the child if the primary complaint is related to respiratory issues. The *Preferred Practice Patterns* indicate that this examination can occur before or after you complete the voice evaluation, but it certainly must occur before any treatment is rendered. Some settings (e.g., school district, hospital) may have established an internal policy that states the evaluation by an otolaryngologist must take place before the child is seen by the SLP for a voice evaluation.

Examination by a physician is necessary for several reasons. It is important that you know as much as possible about the physiology of the pertinent systems (e.g., phonation, respiration, resonation) in order to plan appropriate treatment. In addition, some voice disorders that sound like a "simple hoarseness" may be caused by a serious medical problem such as juvenile papilloma. Treating a child with a serious medical problem without an examination by the physician could result in the child's medical problem getting worse.

In a clinical setting, you have the opportunity to discuss with the parents how important the medical examination is. You may even choose to defer your evaluation until the child has seen the otolaryngologist. There are advantages and disadvantages to scheduling your evaluation before the medical examination. If you see the child before the physician does, you can provide information to the physician about the acoustic and perceptual characteristics of the child's voice. You can also share information about the child's lifestyle and habits that might be contributing to the voice disorder. You can even use the evaluation session to begin to teach some basic vocal hygiene techniques. However, you will not have the benefit of knowing what is wrong with the mechanism, and thus will not be able to provide education about the child's specific problem.

In a school setting, if you cannot easily speak to the parents about the need for the medical evaluation, you might send home an informative letter (See Appendix 2B, page 26) and a fact sheet (See *What Is a Voice Disorder?*, Appendix 2C, page 27) to explain why the medical evaluation is needed. You might also want to include a list of otolaryngologists in the area.

Components of a Clinical Evaluation

When the child is seen for the voice evaluation, it is important that the parents be available to provide information about the child's voice use. If this cannot happen in person, you should speak with the parents by phone before evaluating the child. Ideally the parents will have completed a thorough case history (See Appendix 2D, pages 28-29) prior to the evaluation. Your review of the information on the case history form will allow you to form follow-up questions to ask to gain more information.

Review of case history

The parents' *description of the child's voice* will give you some idea of their awareness of the problem. Information about the *onset of the problem* indicates whether this is a long-standing problem. Some children, for instance, have sounded hoarse since they started talking because they screamed a lot as a baby and may have already developed nodules. The parents may also be able to point to a specific onset (e.g., sounded hoarse after a ball game) that might indicate a problem such as a polyp, which can occur as a result of a single abusive event. A gradual or intermittent onset may indicate a different type of etiology, such as laryngitis.

You can probe for more in-depth information about how the parents think the *voice sounds*, how the child *uses the voice*, and any other *symptoms* related to the voice.

How voice sounds	How child uses voice	Symptoms
hoarse	clears throat	can't sing high notes
breathy	yells/talks loudly	talking makes child tired
voice breaks/cracks	makes funny noises	voice worse in morning
different from peers	talks too softly	voice worse with use
harsh	talks too loudly	tickling/choking sensation
raspy	whispers	frequent burping
	yells when angry	exposed to smoke

Note: This information is listed on the case history form, Appendix 2D, pages 28-29.

You can also probe for any possible psychodynamic issues that may be related to the child's voice problems. These are also listed on the case history form and are drawn from Andrews and Summers 2002:

talks too much aggressive behavior poor self-esteem poor listening skills	doesn't take turns when talking doesn't respond to cues to change behavior always trying to get attention doesn't adapt behavior to the situation

Several *specific medical conditions* are listed that might be related to or causative of the voice problem.

- Asthma – inhaled medications often cause hoarseness
- Allergies – the child may have hoarseness related to the allergies
- Upper respiratory infections/conditions – these may cause the child to cough or clear her throat, resulting in hoarseness
- Gastroesophageal reflux (GERD)/heartburn – if the refluxed material enters the pharynx, it may cause damage to the vocal folds
- Hearing loss – may be the cause of hypofunctional voice patterns with resonance problems
- Frequent laryngitis – may indicate there is an infectious or allergic process that is not controlled; the child may also be causing the laryngitis through vocally abusive behaviors
- Frequent sore throats – may also indicate an infectious or allergic process that is not controlled
- Enlarged tonsils and adenoids – children with enlarged tonsils and adenoids will often have altered resonance because they can't breathe through their noses; these children are typically mouth breathers, this tends to dry the oral and pharyngeal mucosa

Information about *surgeries* may yield information about PE/ventilation tubes for management of otitis media, or even surgery for previous voice problems. If there has been surgery for repair of cleft palate, there may be resonance issues to assess.

Information about *medications* may give information related to the voice disorder. For example, if the child is on allergy medications, perhaps she is experiencing hoarseness related to edema or erythema (redness) of the vocal folds or perhaps she clears her throat frequently in response to allergens. If the child is on medications for asthma, the hoarseness may be tied directly to the use of inhaled medication. Other medications, such as central nervous system stimulants, may have a negative effect on the voice. Some medications for ADD/ADHD are central nervous system stimulants. Antihistamines cause a reduction in secretions and may dry the vocal folds. Anti-cough medications are also mucosal drying agents (Martin 1988). Few children are on medication for GERD, but if you do note such a medication on the case history, it could be informative. In addition, the medication list may indicate problems that could impact the child's participation in therapy. For example, the child's allergy medications may make her drowsy. She may be taking medications for attention deficit, signaling that treatment sessions may need to be modified in length and content.

Information about *hearing acuity* is important because children with reduced hearing may talk loudly. Children with sensori-neural hearing loss may present with resonance problems as a result of altered sensory feedback.

Information about *extra-curricular* activities may shed light on activities during which the child would be prone to abuse her voice. You may also get information about situations in which the child may be using the vocal mechanism inappropriately. For example, you might find the child sings in a chorus and practices several days a week. Perhaps the child is in drama club and speaks in plays without benefit of amplification.

Information about *diet* may be helpful. Beverages (and foods) with *caffeine* can have a drying effect. In addition, if it is suspected that the child has GERD, it will be helpful to know if the child eats foods that precipitate reflux (e.g., spicy foods, citrus, tomatoes).

Evaluation

You can summarize pertinent information from the case history on the *Clinical Voice Evaluation Checklist* (Appendix 2E, pages 30-32). The checklist can also be used to record your observations of the following.

1. Respiration

Adequate respiratory support is necessary for good voice production. The following questions should be answered while listening to the child's spontaneous speech, or during more controlled speech tasks like counting, reciting the alphabet, or reading.

- Does the child appear to inhale adequately to support speech?
- Is there audible inspiration/stridor?
- Does it appear that the child is breathing with the upper chest (i.e., clavicular breathing)?
- Is the child using appropriate phrasing? That is, does she stop and take another breath at the appropriate places or does she seem to talk on low air?

2. Phonation

Andrews and Summers (2002, pp. 151-152) suggested that the following aspects of phonation should be rated as appropriate or inappropriate:

- quality
- onset of voicing
- pitch
- loudness

Terms typically used to describe the *quality* of phonation include *breathy*, *hoarse*, and *harsh*. These are fairly subjective terms and there seems to be little agreement among clinicians about what each means. Fairbanks (1960) was the first to use those three terms. *Breathiness* is perhaps the easiest characteristic to hear. When a voice is breathy, you hear air escaping as the child phonates. Andrews and Summers (2002) reminded us that there can be degrees of breathiness, from a very airy voice to one with only a little breathiness. Breathiness is caused when the margins of the vocal folds are not approximating tightly.

Hoarseness is the most general term used to describe vocal quality. Some researchers state that hoarseness combines breathiness and harshness. *Harshness* indicates that the voice is unpleasant to listen to. There may be more tension with a harsh voice. Sometimes the term *roughness* is used as equivalent to harshness.

You can also note specific abnormalities of quality such as pitch or phonation breaks, loss of voicing, glottal fry (a very low-pitched phonation), or diplophonia (two tones at the same time).

We are interested in the *onset of voicing* because this gives information about the child's use of the vocal mechanism. Voice onset is easiest to hear when the child is saying words that start with a vowel sound. You can use single words or phrases to assess this. Is the onset breathy? Does the child use a hard glottal attack? (See Appendix 8F, page 131, for a list of words, phrases, and sentences that start with a vowel sound.)

Without instrumentation, the assessment of *pitch* is subjective. However, you can determine whether the pitch sounds appropriate for the child's age, gender, and size. You can also model different pitch sounds and see if the child can imitate these. You can assess ability to imitate pitch inflections on sentences too.

For many children, appropriate *loudness* level is part of the voice problem. Does the child's voice sound unusually loud compared to peers and inappropriately loud in certain situations (e.g., Does the child talk very loudly in the library or movie theater?). Can the child control loudness levels when asked?

3. Resonance

If the term *resonance* is used in a narrow way to describe hypernasality, then resonance might be considered an articulation disorder rather than a voice disorder because it is caused by faulty movement and closure of an articulator, the soft palate. However, resonance describes the overall tone of the child's speech and voice. There is a significant interaction between phonation and resonance. The voice (phonation produced at the level of the larynx) is altered by how it resonates throughout all of the supralaryngeal structures. An acceptable voice requires a balance between perceived oral and nasal resonance. Another dichotomy of resonance is that caused by carrying the tongue too far forward or too far back in the oral cavity. If the tongue is held in a high, forward position, the resonance is often described as a thin or baby-sounding voice. Conversely, a tongue carried in the back of the mouth is described as *cul-de-sac resonance*. This may be observed in children who are deaf or may be part of a hyperfunctional voice disorder.

Does the child present with adequate resonance or is the child perceived as hypernasal or hyponasal? Imitation of stimuli with nasal vs. non-nasal sounds can help you make this determination. If the child sounds hypernasal, is it in all contexts or more noticeable in contexts with nasal phonemes, indicating assimilation nasality? Does the child have nasal emission, with air escaping audibly from the nose on pressure consonants? Is the tongue carried too far forward or too far back, affecting the resonance or tone of the voice? Interpretation of nasality should be done cautiously, as some disorders of resonance are caused by structural or physiologic deficits that will need a more thorough, instrumental assessment.

Tips for Discriminating Hypernasality from Hyponasality

Nose Squeeze
Have the child repeat "Many more men on the move" with the nose pinched shut and then without pinching the nose.

Does the child sound stopped up with nose plugged but not when nose released? If so, the child is probably hypernasal.

Does the child sound the same with pinched and unpinched? If so, the child is probably hyponasal.

Nanny Daddy
Have the child repeat "nanny, daddy, nanny, daddy, nanny, daddy"

Do both words sound like "Nanny?" If so, the child is probably hypernasal.

Do both words sound like "Daddy?" If so, the child is probably hyponasal.

Nose Pinch
Have the child sustain the vowel /i/ while you quickly pinch and release the nares.

If the sound of the vowel changes, the child is probably hypernasal.

Counting (may want three trials of each and an average)
With nares open, have the child inhale deeply and then, on exhalation, count as far as possible quickly (2 numbers/second)

Pinch nares shut and repeat. If the child counts further with nares pinched, the child is probably wasting air through the velopharyngeal port and is probably hypernasal.

Adapted from Boone et al. (2005) and Aronson (1990)

---

4. Voice measures

Even without instrumentation, there are several measures you can take to give you more information about the voice.

Pitch Range   Pitch range gives some idea of the flexibility of the voice. A normal range for young, healthy adults is considered to be 2-3 octaves (Bless 1988) and there are considered to be 12 notes to an octave. Sometimes the term *semitones* is used. A semitone is the interval between two adjacent notes. The voice range of boys and girls between the ages of 7 and 10 years is 29 musical semitones (Bohme & Stuchlik 1995).

Maximum Phonation Time   As the child gets older, she can sustain phonation of a vowel sound for longer periods of time. Complete normative data is not available, but Launer (1971) reported that by age 9, girls can sustain vowels for about 8 seconds and boys for 11 seconds. By age 12, each can sustain a vowel for 12 seconds. Inability to do this may indicate trouble with closure of the glottis or poor respiratory support. Reduced maximum phonation time is also seen in children with velopharyngeal insufficiency, with air escaping out the nose.

s/z ratio   The *s/z* ratio can be used as a tool to judge vocal quality. The theory is that if the vocal folds are vibrating normally, the child should be able to sustain both the voiceless /s/ and the voiced /z/ sounds an equal number of seconds. The ratio, then, would be one-to-one (1.0). If the ratio is greater than 1.4, the child may have some vibratory dysfunction of the vocal folds.

Example of *s/z* ratio

Child sustains /s/ for 12 seconds and /z/ for 11 seconds
12 divided by 11 = 1.09 (within normal limits)

Child sustains /s/ for 17 seconds and /z/ for 10 seconds
17 divided by 10 = 1.7 (abnormal limits)

Perceptual checklists

In addition to (or instead of) the *Clinical Voice Evaluation Checklist* (Appendix 2E, pages 30-32), you may want to use a perceptual checklist that rates severity of characteristics to record your observations about the child's voice. The *Consensus Auditory Perceptual Evaluation of Voice (CAPE-V)*, developed by ASHA Special Interest Division 3 (Voice Disorders), includes the voice characteristics of roughness, breathiness, strain, pitch, and loudness. The checklist allows you to rate each of these as mild, moderate, or severe and to indicate if the characteristic is consistently or intermittently observed. The checklist and its description, instructions, and scoring can be found online at *www.asha.org/about/membership-certification/divs/div_3.htm* (scroll down the page to find the *CAPE-V*). Another checklist, the *Voice Rating Severity Scale*, is included in *The Boone Voice Program for Children* (Boone 1993). It is a 7-point scale that rates characteristics such as pitch, loudness, quality, resonance, rate, and range. Wilson (1970) designed the *Voice Profile* which includes a severity rating and descriptions of pitch and resonance as well as range.

Although perceptual checklists can help organize the information being collected about the child's voice, most scales used in this way have been shown to have very poor reliability, particularly in the middle of the scales. That is, raters are more reliable when rating a severe problem than they are when they are rating voice problems on the mild to moderate end of the scale (Kreiman & Gerratt 1998).

ASHA NOMS

The ASHA *National Outcomes Measurement System* (NOMS) is a database for collection of outcomes information. There is a pre-K component for children ages 3-5 and a K-12 component that can be used in the schools. Each contains a 7-point scale, called a *Functional Communication Measure* (FCM) for voice. There are also FCMs for many other aspects of communication disorders (e.g., receptive language, expressive language, articulation/phonology). Participation in the NOMS allows the clinician to rate the child's voice at the beginning of intervention and again at the end of intervention. This functional rating scale is written in terms that teachers, parents, and other non-SLPs can understand. The information from your program can be compared to national data from similar programs. This allows you to make prognoses, estimate length of treatment, etc. For more information on NOMS, contact ASHA: *www.asha.org/members/research/NOMS*

23

Ability to modify behaviors

Assessing the child's ability to modify any abnormal respiratory, phonatory, and resonatory behaviors is similar to stimulability testing with a child who has an articulation disorder. Determining how easily the child can change these behaviors will help you plan treatment and determine a prognosis.

Impact of voice disorder

What impact does the voice disorder have on the child's participation in activities at school, at home, and in the community? Is the impact consistently observed or is it more noticeable in certain situations? Has the child limited participation in some activities because of the problem? How much impact the voice disorder is having may play a large part in determining how motivated the child is to address the problem. If the child is not willing to change behaviors, there is little hope for making a substantial change in vocal characteristics.

Writing the report

Depending on the setting in which you work, you may generate a typed report or a handwritten note to summarize your findings. A template for your summary report is included in Appendix 2F, page 33. Appendix 2G (page 34) is a listing of International Classification of Diseases, Ninth Revision, Clinical Modification (ICD-9-CM) Codes that can be used when writing your report.

Summary

The clinical evaluation of the child's voice disorder consists of gathering information about the child's medical history and voice use. It also includes careful observation of the child's vocal behaviors with information about how voice use changes in different settings. The child's ability to modify these behaviors and the impact the voice disorder is having on the child's participation in school, home, and play activities will help determine the child's willingness to change behaviors. All of this information will form the basis for your intervention. Your evaluation can provide useful information to the physician who will examine the child's larynx (if your evaluation was completed before referral). The clinical findings may be combined with instrumental results if an instrumental exam is performed to further enhance your treatment plan.

Observation of Child's Voice Use

Child's Name _____

Date Completed _____

Completed by   ___   Classroom teacher

              ___   Other teacher (specify: _____)

              ___   Coach (specify: _____)

              ___   Parent(s)

              ___   Other (specify: _____)

Please check all that apply.

☐   1. Talks louder than other children in the classroom

☐   2. Talks to children at far side of classroom instead of going over to children

☐   3. Yells on the playground more than other children

☐   4. Makes funny noises with voice (e.g., truck sounds, character voices)

☐   5. Yells up and down the stairs

☐   6. Yells to call pets

☐   7. Cries loudly when upset

☐   8. Uses voice to express anger (e.g., yells at siblings, raises voice to peers)

☐   9. Yells during sports (either as spectator or participant)

☐   10. Coughs/clears throat a lot

Comments

_____

_____

_____

_____

Complete and return by _____ to _____.

Speech-Language Pathologist

To: Parents of _____

From: _____
                    Speech-Language Pathologist

Re: Voice problem

Date: _____

Through screening/referral from your child's teacher, your child has been identified as having a voice disorder. Your child's voice sounds:

_____

_____

Before I can do an evaluation and therapy, your child needs to be seen by an otolaryngologist (Ear, Nose, and Throat doctor) to examine your child's vocal folds. This examination is necessary to find out what might be causing the voice problem and to make sure we are not overlooking a serious medical problem. I have included a fact sheet about common voice disorders in children and a list of doctors in our area.

Please call me if you have questions about taking your child to the doctor. Please take this letter with you when you take your child to the doctor and ask the doctor to send a copy of his/her report to me at _____. As soon as I receive that report, I will set up a meeting to discuss the physician's findings with you and to ask permission to evaluate your child's voice.

Also, I would appreciate it if you would complete the enclosed *Case History* questionnaire and *Observation of Child's Voice Use* form and bring them along when we meet.

Please feel free to call me with any questions at _____.

Thank you.

Enclosures
- *What Is a Voice Disorder?* fact sheet (Appendix 2C)
- List of Ear, Nose, and Throat doctors in our area
- *Case History* questionnaire (Appendix 2D)
- *Observation of Child's Voice Use* (Appendix 2A)

What Is a Voice Disorder?

Why is the voice important?

A healthy voice is essential for participation in school and extra-curricular activities. Children use their voices to answer questions in class, express emotions, and interact with their friends.

How is voice produced?

Voice is produced by vibration of the vocal folds. These are small muscles inside the larynx, or voice box. Air from the lungs travels over the vocal folds causing vibration. The sound from the vibration travels through the throat, nose, and mouth. The sound is modified as it travels through the throat, nose, and mouth, and these changes determine what the voice will sound like.

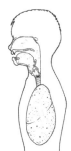

What is a voice disorder?

A voice that sounds significantly different from other children the same age and gender may be disordered. A voice can be hoarse or harsh. The pitch may be too high or too low. The child may have to use too much effort to talk. The child may lose his/her voice after a lot of talking, or be unable to raise the volume of his/her voice. A voice that sounds nasal (sounding like the speech is coming from the child's nose), is sometimes related to a voice problem.

What are some causes of voice disorders?

The most common cause of vocal problems is vocal misuse and abuse. Anyone who uses his/her voice excessively may develop related voice problems. Children in particular may yell and scream, talk too loudly, and make strange noises with their voices as they play. Misuse may include talking without good breathing support or talking at too high or too low a pitch. These misuses and abuses may result in changes to the vocal folds. These changes might include swelling or even growths on the vocal folds. Other causes of voice disorders include upper respiratory infections, acid reflux, and growths on the vocal folds caused by viral infection instead of by abuse.

How do I find out if there is something wrong with my child's larynx (voice box)?

Have your child examined by an otolaryngologist (also called an ENT or throat doctor). The doctor can look at the vocal folds and determine if there is anything wrong with the vocal folds.

Why does my child need to see the ENT doctor?

Some childhood voice problems are caused by physical problems that need medical or even surgical intervention. This is unlikely, but the speech-language pathologist (SLP) cannot proceed with an evaluation and treatment of the voice disorder until a medical doctor has given clearance that it is all right to do so.

How are voice disorders treated?

Some voice disorders may need medical or surgical intervention. However, most problems are treated through therapy provided by an SLP. An SLP will help your child understand what the child has been doing with his/her voice that has caused the problem. The SLP will work closely with your child and you (the child's parents) to modify those behaviors and to teach the child better ways to use his/her voice. In addition, your child may learn specific exercises to improve breathing and sound production.

Appendix 2C
The Source for Children's Voice Disorders

27

Copyright © 2005 LinguiSystems, Inc.

Case History

Child's Name _____ Child's Birthdate _____

Person Completing Form_____ Today's Date _____

Relationship to Child _____

Please describe your child's voice.

_____

_____

How long has your child's voice sounded this way? _____

Did the voice problem come on slowly or suddenly? _____

Check all that describe your child's voice.

_____ hoarse	_____ frequently whispers
_____ breathy	_____ deals with anger by yelling
_____ voice breaks/cracks	_____ can't sing high notes
_____ harsh	_____ complains that talking makes him/her tired
_____ raspy	_____ voice worse in morning
_____ frequently clears throat	_____ voice worse with use
_____ frequently yells/talks loudly	_____ complains of tickling/choking sensation
_____ frequently makes funny noises	_____ frequent burping
_____ talks too softly	_____ exposed to smoke
_____ talks too loudly	_____ voice sounds different from peers

Check all interpersonal skills your child exhibits.

_____ talks too much	_____ doesn't take turns when talking
_____ aggressive behavior	_____ doesn't respond to cues to change behavior
_____ poor self-esteem	_____ always trying to get attention
_____ poor listening skills	_____ doesn't adapt behavior to situation

Medical Conditions

Does your child have now, or have a history of, any of the following?
(Please provide more information on those you mark *yes*.)

yes / no   asthma _____

yes / no   allergies _____

yes / no   upper respiratory infections/conditions _____

yes / no   gastroesophageal reflux (GERD)/heartburn _____

yes / no   hearing loss _____

yes / no   frequent laryngitis _____

yes / no   frequent sore throats _____

yes / no   enlarged tonsils and adenoids _____

yes / no   other medical conditions _____

Has your child had any surgeries?   yes   no   If *yes*, please list: _____

Medications

List any medications your child takes and what the medication is for:

                 Medication   For

_____   _____

_____   _____

_____   _____

Hearing Acuity

When was the last time your child's hearing was tested?_____

What were results of that evaluation?_____

Has your child been examined by an Ear, Nose, and Throat doctor?   yes   no

If *yes*, please list date(s) seen and the name and address of doctor(s):

_____

_____

_____

Please contact the doctor(s) and ask that a copy of each evaluation be sent to us.

Extra-Curricular Activities

What extra-curricular activities is your child involved in?

_____

_____

_____

How often does he/she participate in these activities?

_____

_____

_____

Diet

How often does your child drink beverages with caffeine (e.g., cola)?

_____ never

_____ occasionally (1-3 per week)

_____ has at least one every day

_____ has more than one every day

Appendix 2D, *continued*
The Source for Children's Voice Disorders
    29

Clinical Voice Evaluation Checklist

Client _____   Client Birthdate _____

Date of Evaluation _____

Reason for referral _____

_____

History of problems _____

Medical history related to problem _____

_____

Respiration	Desired behaviors are listed in bold.

yes/no	**breathes adequately to support speech**
yes/no	talks on low air
yes/no	breathes with upper chest (clavicular)
yes/no	**breathes with diaphragm (abdomen)**
yes/no	noisy inhalation (stridor)

Sustains: /a/   yes/no   /i/   yes/no

Phonation Quality

Quality in spontaneous speech sounds:

yes/no	**appropriate**
yes/no	breathy
yes/no	harsh
yes/no	hoarse

The following abnormalities were noted:

yes/no	phonation breaks within a word
yes/no	pitch breaks (indicate if pitch breaks up or down)
yes/no	loss of voice on more than one word
yes/no	glottal fry
yes/no	diplophonia

continued on next page

Onset of phonation

On vowel initiate words (e.g. *arm, out, each, itch*)

yes/no   **appropriate**

yes/no   breathy

yes/no   hard attack

On sentences beginning with vowels (*Aunt Emma ate it all. Is everyone already eating?*)

yes/no   **appropriate**

yes/no   breathy

yes/no   hard attack

Pitch

In spontaneous speech, habitual pitch:

yes/no   **appropriate for age and sex**

yes/no   too high compared to age/gender peers

yes/no   too low compared to age/gender peers

yes/no   starts utterance with adequate pitch but drops too low at end

yes/no   **can initiate sentences at appropriate pitch**

yes/no   **uses good inflection in voice**

Loudness

Loudness level

yes/no   **appropriate for 1 on 1 setting**

yes/no   too loud

yes/no   too soft

Can demonstrate control of loudness

yes/no   **can count 1-5 soft to loud, getting a little louder on each number**

Can imitate three levels of loudness

yes/no   **library voice (not a whisper)**

yes/no   **classroom voice**

yes/no   **auditorium voice**

continued on next page

Resonance

Desired behaviors are listed in bold.

yes/no	**appropriate balance between oral and nasal resonance**
yes/no	Does spontaneous speech sound hypernasal?
yes/no	Does spontaneous speech sound hyponasal?
yes/no	Is the child perceived as nasal only in nasal contexts? (*Many men made much noise.* vs. *All babies do is play.*)
yes/no	**tongue carriage appropriate**
yes/no	tongue carried too far forward
yes/no	tongue carried too far back (cul de sac)

Voice Measures

Pitch range _____ number of notes child can produce (at least 20)

Maximum phonation time

/a/ _____ seconds

/i/ _____ seconds

s/z ratio   s_____ (seconds)/z_____ (seconds) = _____ ratio (abnormal if greater than 1)

Ability to modify behaviors (If any abnormal behaviors are noted, describe child's ability to modify.)

Respiration _____

Phonation _____

Quality _____

Onset _____

Pitch _____

Loudness _____

Resonance _____

Summary Template for Voice Evaluation

Child's Name _____   Date of Evaluation _____

Birthdate _____   Age _____

Parent(s) _____   Physician _____

Address _____   Referral Source _____

Phone _____

___

Reason for referral _____

History of problem _____

Medical problems related to voice problem _____

_____

Observations of respiratory support for speech _____

_____

Observations of phonation

    Quality _____

    Onset of phonation _____

    Pitch _____

    Loudness _____

Observations of resonance _____

Voice measures

    Pitch range _____

    Maximum phonation time _____

    s/z ratio _____

Child's ability to modify behaviors _____

Diagnosis _____

_____

ICD-9-CM code(s) _____

Prognosis for changing vocal behaviors _____

_____

Recommendations _____

_____

ICD-9-CM Codes

Use a code that describes the vocal characteristics. Include any known medical diagnoses. You can list one as secondary to the other (e.g., hoarseness [784.49] secondary to vocal nodules [478.5]).

ICD Diagnostic Codes for Problems SLPs Treat	
Code	**Description**
300.11	Conversion disorder
306.1	Respiratory (psychogenic cough)
784.4	Voice disturbance
784.40	Voice disturbance, unspecified
784.41	Aphonia (loss of voice)
784.49	Voice disturbance, other (change in voice, dysphonia, hoarseness, hypernasality, hyponasality)
786.2	Cough

ICD Diagnostic Codes for Related Medical Problems	
Code	**Description**
464.0	Acute laryngitis
476.0	Chronic laryngitis
478.3	Paralysis of vocal cords or larynx
478.31	Unilateral, partial
478.32	Unilateral, complete
478.33	Bilateral, partial
478.34	Bilateral, complete
478.4	Polyp of vocal cords or larynx
478.5	Other disease of vocal cords
478.6	Edema of larynx
478.75	Laryngeal spasms
478.79	Unspecified disease of the larynx (other)
530.81	Gastroesophageal reflux (GERD)

In addition to ICD-9 diagnostic codes, you may also need to use CPT codes for billing, such as the following:

92506	Evaluation of speech, language, voice, communication, and/or auditory processing
92507	Treatment of speech, language, voice, communication, and/or auditory processing disorder; individual
92512	Nasal function studies
92520	Laryngeal function studies

International Classification of Diseases, Ninth Revision, Clinical Modification. (2004). American Medical Association, Ingenix, Inc.
Current Procedural Terminology CPT 2005 Professional Edition. (2004). American Medical Association. Chicago, IL: AMA Press.

3 Instrumental Evaluation of Voice

Most SLPs do not work in a setting that allows for the use of sophisticated equipment for voice assessment. However, this situation should not prevent you from evaluating voice through analysis of perceptual voice quality, case history, and specific behaviors. No instrumental measure can take the place of clinical judgment used to interpret perceptual analysis, case history information, and observation of behaviors. In fact, sometimes information obtained during an instrumental evaluation does not match what is heard. In this case, you will need to determine how to rectify this mismatch of information.

Instrumentation provides additional information in order to make inferences about underlying vocal fold physiology. Lack of instrumentation is sometimes frustrating as instrumental measurements can add important information to the understanding of what is happening with the respiratory, phonatory, and resonatory mechanisms. During treatment, instrumentation can provide feedback to both you and the client, and the objective measures obtained from instrumentation can demonstrate progress being made in treatment (e.g., pre- and post- test numerical values on some of the measures).

Even if you don't use sophisticated equipment during your evaluations, you should understand the information such equipment can provide. This knowledge will help you determine when to make a referral to a clinic that can perform instrumental assessment. It will also help you understand reports you receive from such a clinic. The information in this chapter is not intended to prepare you to perform instrumental evaluations. It provides an overview of the kinds of instrumental measures obtained during an evaluation and describe equipment used to gather this information. Only measures that are used clinically, as opposed to research labs, will be described in detail. If you intend to use instrumentation, it is important to seek out much more detailed information so that you understand the physiology and theory related to instrumental measures.

Instrumental analysis of voice obtains objective measures that might be broken down into three main categories:

1. Analyzing the acoustic signal

2. Measuring aerodynamic changes in pressure or flow

3. Recording visual images of vocal fold vibration

Additional measurements (e.g., electroglottography [EGG], electromyography [EMG]) are also considered part of the instrumental evaluation. Different equipment is used to capture these different pieces of information, which is then interpreted.

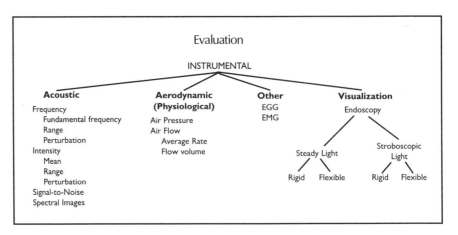

Acoustic Measures

Acoustic measures reflect the complex interaction between the air stream from the respiratory system, the movement in the larynx, and the modification of the acoustic signal in the supralaryngeal cavities. The basic features of the acoustics of voice that can be measured are described by Stemple et al. (2000).

- *Frequency* is an acoustic measure of the perceptual judgment of pitch.
- *Intensity* is an acoustic measure of the perceptual judgment of loudness.
- *Perturbation measures* assess the amount of variation from cycle to cycle in the acoustic signal (either frequency or amplitude of the waveform being analyzed).
- *Ratio of signal-to-noise* can also be called *harmonic energy to noise*. This measure reflects the ratio of periodic to aperiodic (i.e., noisy) components of the signal.
- *Spectral features* provide information about how the supraglottic vocal tract contributes to the voice signal. These are obtained through acoustic techniques that create visual displays, providing information about fundamental frequency and harmonic energies in sound.

Some of these measures can discriminate normal from abnormal vocal quality. A few have standardized information against which the values can be compared. This is not a perfect science, and there are disagreements between what the voice sounds like and what the instrumentation shows. Some voices are so impaired (e.g., the child can't produce a sustained voice) that a reliable acoustic analysis cannot be done. None of the measures can tell what impaired physiology or function is causing the voice problem, although some inferences can be made. Additionally, there is a lack of normative data for children (Harvey 1996).

Frequency

Frequency measures include mean fundamental frequency, frequency range, and the perturbation ratings.

Fundamental frequency

Fundamental frequency is how fast the vocal folds are vibrating and is indicated in Hertz (Hz) or cycles per second. Fundamental frequency may be abbreviated Fo. When we listen to the child's voice, fundamental frequency is perceived as pitch.

The child speaks into a microphone connected to the instrument. The fundamental frequency may be obtained by having the child produce a vowel sound and hold it. Fundamental frequency is also obtained from a connected speech sample. Multiple trials are typical as fundamental frequency can vary according to the speech task and the intensity.

The instrumentation shows the frequency pattern on a screen and then computes an average fundamental frequency. By looking at the screen, you can observe intonation patterns in the voice. For instance, if the child speaks in what seems like a monotone, the tracing on the screen will seem relatively flat. If the child uses good intonation, there will be variability in the tracing.

What is typical for a child? Recall that there is limited normative data for pediatrics. The following data were obtained as children age 6-10 produced a sustained /a/ sound.

	Mean	Minimum	Maximum
Boys	226 Hz	179 Hz	272 Hz
Girls	238 Hz	193 Hz	294 Hz

From Glaze et al. (1988). Boone et al. (2005) indicate that the typical child's voice is between 262 to 294 Hz.

Frequency range

When assessing fundamental frequency (pitch), measures of pitch range are usually obtained. *Range* is the difference between the highest note and lowest note (i.e., pitch) the child can produce. The range is an indicator of the capabilities of the larynx (Andrews and Summers 2002). It is achieved by asking the client to produce the lowest note possible and then move up the scale with a continuous tone to the highest note possible. A change in fundamental frequency range (e.g., the client now can go higher or start lower) may indicate an improvement in the vocal mechanism. For example, as the client's vocal nodules resolve, you might observe a greater pitch range.

Perturbation

Perturbation is sometimes described as the amount of "roughness" in the voice. Acoustically it is the cycle-to-cycle variability in a signal. This measure can only be obtained while the client produces a sustained vowel. If the measure were taken during a speech sample, the instrument would perceive the breaks between words as abnormal phonation breaks and would provide a faulty analysis.

There are two terms commonly used to describe perturbation, one for frequency and one for intensity. The amount of perturbation in frequency (perceived as pitch) is called *jitter*. See the next page for an explanation of perturbation in amplitude (perceived as loudness) called *shimmer*.

There are many factors that can interfere with obtaining an accurate rating of perturbation because many things can contribute to vocal instability. That is, a particular perturbation rating does not signify a certain problem with the voice. These measures can help demonstrate improvement in vocal quality when used during the course of treatment.

Intensity

Vocal intensity is the acoustic term for what we perceive as loudness. Vocal intensity is abbreviated Io. It is measured in decibels (dB). There are some challenges to collecting intensity data because it can be affected by background noise, the kind of task the client is completing, and even the distance between the microphone and the mouth.

Mean or habitual intensity

Talking too loudly, at least in some situations, is a common problem in children. Therefore, measuring intensity levels is important. Measures are usually taken on sustained vowels and in connected speech. Intensity measures can be taken with a simple sound meter.

As expected, normative information about intensity levels varies according to the task and the situation in which the data was obtained. Children age 6-10, when producing /a/, showed this mean and range.

	Mean	Range
Children 6-10	70 dB	60-99 dB

From Glaze et al. (1990). Boone et al. (2005) indicate that 45-65 dB would be average for a child.

Intensity range

Intensity range is a reflection of how quietly and how loudly the child can phonate. Typical tasks include asking the child to produce a vowel sound at the softest level and then shouting "Hey" as loud as possible. As with most acoustic measures, multiple trials are used.

Perturbation Measures

The cycle-to-cycle variability in intensity is also a reflection of the roughness in the voice. This type of perturbation is called *shimmer*. Remember that it is obtained only on a sustained vowel. There is no good normative data on perturbation at this time, and if a client shows a decrease in perturbation, it is difficult to impossible to determine what has contributed to this decrease (Stemple et al. 2000).

The relationship between frequency, intensity, and perturbation

Keep in mind the relationship between frequency and intensity. Typically frequency goes up with increased intensity. That is, when the client produces a higher note, he also gets louder. There is also a relationship between perturbation and fundamental frequency, with the former decreasing as the latter increases. That is, there is less perturbation at higher pitches. These values also change depending on the stimuli.

Signal-to-noise ratios

These ratios are determined by the instrumentation through the use of specific formulae. The greater the signal or harmonic energy (good signal coming from the voice) compared to noise energy indicates better vocal function. This measure is used mostly to show progress from one session to the next. There are no absolute values of what is or isn't normal.

Spectral images

These three-dimensional spectral images aren't used much clinically. The images show the influence of both the sound made at the level of the glottis and the effect on that sound by the supraglottic structures. Clinical interpretations can be made from the spectrogram. For example, changes in vocal quality can lead to increased noise in the spectrogram (Yanagihara 1967).

Aerodynamic (Physiologic) Measures

Aerodynamic measures have been used to discriminate normal from abnormal vocal fold function, describe severity, and possibly help distinguish etiology (Andrews and Summers 2002). Two aerodynamic measures are often used to provide information about the ability of the larynx to valve, or control, the airflow from the lungs. These are *measures of flow* (how much air is flowing across the larynx) and *pressure* (how much pressure is exerted by that air on the vocal folds). These measures are called:

- subglottic pressure
- transglottic flow
    - ⇨ average flow rate
    - ⇨ flow volume

These measures of the relationship between pressure and flow relate more closely to the vocal fold valving function and therefore are sometimes called *physiologic measures* (as compared to the acoustic measures previously described).

Subglottic pressure

Adequate subglottal pressure is necessary to produce voice. It is typically measured by determining pressure in the oral cavity on a plosive. It is then estimated that this would be the same pressure found subglottally. If subglottic pressures are high, you might presume that the client has a tight glottis, as in hyperfunction. This measure is not often taken with children because they have trouble with the tube that is placed in the mouth.

Airflow rate and volume

Instrumentation for analysis of these measures during speech captures the airflow as the client speaks into a mask. Typically the client is asked to sustain a vowel sound while the measures of average airflow rate and flow volume are obtained. These measures can yield some information about the glottis. For example, if the average air flow rate is faster than typical, it might indicate that the glottis isn't closing well—thus allowing the air to escape too quickly. A client with a hyperfunctional voice pattern will demonstrate reduced airflow rates. On the other hand, if there is excess subglottic pressure, the client may be exhibiting hyperfunctional voice use; that is, squeezing the larynx so tightly that air pressure builds up under the vocal folds. Normative data continues to be investigated.

Other Physiologic Measures

There are several other physiologic measures that provide related information about vocal fold movement. Electromyography can be done with needles (this is invasive and is done by a physician) or surface electrodes. Inverse filtering, another technique, is not used clinically. One other common measure, electroglottography (EGG), is used clinically. EGG is a non-invasive technique that uses two electrodes placed on either side of the thyroid cartilage. It is a measure of relative glottal contact. It produces a waveform that can be used to interpret vocal fold vibratory behavior. It is particularly appropriate for the pediatric population because of its non-invasiveness, relatively low cost, and ease of use (Cheyne et al. 1999).

Visualization

Visualization of the larynx is done on a basic level by an otolaryngologist during an indirect examination of the larynx with a laryngeal mirror. The availability of endoscopy has made more sophisticated visualization of the larynx commonplace, and an important part of the diagnosis of voice disorders. ASHA considers "that vocal tract visualization and imaging for the purpose of diagnosing and treating patients with voice or resonance/aeromechanical disorders is within the scope of practice of the speech-language pathologist" (ASHA 2004). ASHA (1998) also recognizes, in a joint position statement with the American Academy of Otolaryngology, that "Physicians are the only professionals qualified and licensed to render medical diagnoses related to the identification of laryngeal pathology as it affects voice."

Kinds of lights used with endoscopy

Two kinds of light are used with a fiberoptic endoscope to visualize the larynx: steady state and stroboscopic.

Steady state light is produced by a halogen bulb. It allows visualization of anatomic structures and basic vocal fold function, providing information similar to that obtained in an indirect examination of the larynx.

Stroboscopic light is used to observe the vibratory patterns of the vocal folds. It is produced by a steady halogen bulb and a flashing xenon light. This type of light is needed because the vocal folds vibrate much too fast for the movement to be seen by the naked eye (60 to 1400 Hz). Stroboscopic light sends out pulses of light that are timed to the frequency of the child's voice. The camera is basically recording multiple "still" pictures that appear to our eye to be pictures moving in slow motion. Have you ever seen little books where each page contains a drawing that is slightly different, and when you fan through the pages, the images look like they are moving? That is essentially what stroboscopy is doing when capturing images of the vocal folds in action.

Stroboscopic examination allows you to see:
- mass lesions
- nature of vocal fold margins (smooth or rough)
- symmetry of movement
- regularity of movement
- patterns of glottal closure
- amplitude of vibration
- presence or absence of mucosal wave (Stemple et al. 2000, p. 170)

Types of scopes used with steady state and stroboscopic light

Two types of scopes can be used with either type of light. The flexible scope is inserted transnasally while the rigid scope is inserted into the mouth. Each offers some advantages and many voice clinicians use both within the same exam to gather different information.

Advantage	Rigid scope	Flexible scope
No gag		X
Larger and clearer picture	X	
Closer to larynx for better image	X	
No restriction on tongue and jaw		X
Used with continuous speech samples		X
Allows view of velopharyngeal mechanism		X
May cause less anxiety in children	X	
Same size scope for adults or children	X	
Better view of vocal fold vibratory patterns	X	

When is stroboscopy indicated?

Stemple et al. (2000) provide a list of conservative indications for stroboscopy:

- persistent dysphonia (greater than 3 weeks) that can't be explained with other visualization techniques
- professional voice users with deterioration in their performance
- before surgery on larynx
- clarify etiology of disorder
- determine optimal management plan

Summary

Instrumentation can add significant information to the evaluation of voice disorders but does not replace your clinical evaluation and judgment. If you provide services in a setting that does not have instrumentation such as described in this chapter, familiarize yourself with facilities near you that do. Work in collaboration with those professionals (e.g., ENT, SLP) to ensure the child receives a comprehensive workup of the voice disorder.

4 | Planning and Implementing Intervention

After you gather information from the clinical exam, from any instrumental examinations, and from any pertinent medical examinations, it is time to plan treatment. Planning voice therapy for a preteen child presents many challenges. This chapter is designed to help you think through these challenges and plan your course of intervention. The chapter also provides you with sample forms and a master list of long-term goals, short-term goals, and treatment objectives that may be helpful. Subsequent chapters will provide in-depth information about particular treatment techniques.

Integrating Evaluation Information

The clinical evaluation

The clinical evaluation provides information about how the child uses her voice in a variety of situations. As a result of the evaluation, you also gain important information about the parents' views (and other significant adults' views) concerning the child's voice disorder. You have considered what impact any related medical disorders may be having on the child's voice. You have an understanding about the level of awareness the child has about her voice disorder and whether or not she is motivated to address the problem. You have also determined whether the child is stimulable to make changes in the aspects of her voice that need to be changed. And you have gained information about any psychodynamic issues that might be provoking or contributing to the use of vocally abusive behaviors.

The medical evaluation

The medical evaluation, conducted most often by an otolaryngologist (ENT), provides information about any abnormalities of the vocal mechanism itself. If structural abnormalities such as vocal nodules were identified, the physician has probably recommended whether surgical intervention is indicated at this time. If surgical intervention has been suggested, you'll need to adjust the timing of your intervention. Does the physician want you to try voice therapy first before a final determination is made about such surgical intervention? Or does the physician intend to perform surgery and have you see the child for voice therapy after the surgery? If the latter is the case, you need to find out exactly how long after surgery the physician will say the child can begin therapy. The medical evaluation may have revealed that a medical problem was causing or significantly contributing to the voice disorder. Perhaps the physician observed signs of damage to the vocal folds associated with gastroesophageal reflux (GERD). Or perhaps the physician determined that inhaled corticosteroids (which the child uses for treatment of her asthma) are largely to blame for the voice quality. If such medically-related problems are determined to be contributing to the problem, you'll need to decide whether to begin therapy or to wait and see if any changes in medical management have significant impact on the voice disorder.

Medical evaluation may also have indicated that there were no structural abnormalities, but that the voice problem is a result of misuse of the mechanism.

Perhaps the physician observed some hyperfunctional vocal behaviors during the examination. If that is the case, hopefully a more complete instrumental examination of the voice was completed. If not, you may want to request that one be done.

The instrumental voice evaluation

The instrumental voice evaluation may include acoustic and aerodynamic (physiologic) measures in addition to visualization of the larynx with steady light or stroboscopic light. These findings provide much more detailed information about what the child is doing with the larynx which will be very helpful in planning appropriate treatment. Such an instrumental evaluation is usually completed by an SLP working in an otolaryngologist's office or specialized voice clinic. In less than optimal situations, the otolaryngologist may conduct the evaluation without the SLP. (See Chapter 3, pages 35-41, for more information.)

Gaining Support for Voice Treatment

Helping the child understand the problem

There is a significant difference in providing voice therapy for a preteen child compared to treating a motivated adolescent or adult. The adolescent or adult who ends up in your office realizes the significance of the voice disorder and has decided to do something about it. The young child, on the other hand, is probably being seen because an adult in her life has decided that there's something wrong with her voice.

The child will need a basic explanation of the relationship between the respiratory, phonatory, and resonance systems. (See Appendix 4A, page 54.) With a young child, you may have to adjust the way you talk about these systems and the problems so that the child can understand. You may have to use analogies like the ones below that make sense for the child's developmental age.

Andrews and Summers (2002) point out how important it is that the concepts being discussed are made concrete for the child. They suggest using the term *different* when describing the child's voice rather than using negative terms like *wrong* or *bad*. They also caution that you should not use the same term to describe two different parameters of the child's voice. For example if you use the word *low* to describe a target volume, you should not use the word *low* to describe an inappropriately low pitch.

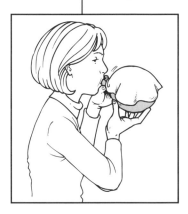

Using hands-on props can help the young child understand your message. An inflated balloon is a good stand-in for the lungs. Blowing up the balloon can help the child see how the lungs fill with air. You can put a lightweight cloth or paper towel on top of the balloon to help the child understand how we can "see" the lungs inflate by watching movement of the abdominal wall rise and fall. Blow some air in and then let a little escape to demonstrate movement.

If you pinch and stretch the top of the inflated balloon and slowly release it to let the air come out, it can help the child understand how the air from the lungs moves through the vocal folds to make sound.

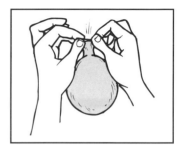

Different sizes of rubber bands can also help the child understand how vocal folds can become swollen and to understand the difference in the sound that is produced when vocal folds become thicker. Stretch a thin rubber band between your fingers and "pluck" it. Do the same with a thick rubber band. Help the child hear the difference in the sounds made.

It's also important for the child to understand the relationship between respiration and phonation and the important role that air from the lungs plays in vibrating (moving) the vocal folds. A cube of Jell-O makes a nice prop for demonstrating quick vibratory movement. Jostle the Jell-O with a spoon as you explain to the child that air from the lungs makes the vocal folds vibrate similarly to the jiggly movement observed in the Jell-O.

The child also needs to understand that the way she is using her voice is causing some of the problems. You may need to demonstrate for the child some of the abnormal behaviors contrasted with normal use of these different systems. Cartoon or fictional characters with different vocal types can help illustrate abnormal and/or target behaviors (e.g., Bugs Bunny has a nasal resonance, Darth Vader has a deep pitch).

The child needs to understand that psychodynamic factors, including interpersonal skills, may play a large part in the voice problem. If the child is aggressive, for example, she is likely to use a loud voice in many situations. Her muscles may be very tense. If the child has a habit of ignoring feedback, you will need to discuss how this behavior will have an impact on changing her voice. If the child's pattern is to constantly seek attention, you'll need to point out that she is doing this now by using her voice in inappropriate and harmful ways.

Motivating the child to change

Helping the child understand how the mechanism works and how to change the use of the mechanism is the easy part. The hard part is motivating the child to want to do something about the problem. Unless the child is totally aphonic or dysphonic to the point of being unable to participate in desired activities, she is probably not very motivated to make a change in how she is communicating. It is very difficult for children to understand a long-term impact. Consider the following examples:

- Explaining to a 10-year-old that her hoarse vocal quality will make it impossible for her to sing in the chorus in high school has absolutely no relevance to the child.

- Telling a child that his very loud volume is annoying to his teacher will fall on deaf ears if this loud volume helps him get what he wants on the playground.

- Convincing a child that the strange sounds he makes with his voice are damaging his vocal folds will have little impact when classmates reinforce him because they think the sounds are funny.

It is likely that the child will only be motivated to change if she understands how the target behaviors will help her get what she wants. The child needs to understand that the changes you are requesting will be beneficial in day-to-day situations.

Helping the child understand the relationship between emotions, behaviors, and the voice

At different ages, children have very different understandings of what emotions are, how they are perceived, and how to appropriately demonstrate emotions. Andrews and Summers (2002) summarize the work of several researchers by indicating that there may be two main stages of children's knowledge of emotion.

Stage I: Younger than 6 years of age

A young child judges emotion by the situation and her own reaction. The child sees the effects of emotion in simple positive and negative terms and makes no attempt to explain them. This pattern continues until sometime between the ages of 6 and 11 when the child moves to a more advanced stage of understanding.

Stage II: 11 years and older

An older child judges emotion not only by the situation and her reaction, but also by the reactions of others and her own inner mental state.

An understanding of these developmental stages is important as you talk with the child and help her try to change the way she uses her voice to deal with emotions. Some children with voice disorders may have difficulty with interpersonal relationships, making it particularly challenging to deal with the emotional component of the voice disorder.

Utilizing a Behavior Change Reinforcement System

You may need to use tangible reinforcers for the child. These may be used immediately to reinforce target vocal behaviors or to reinforce the child for not using an abusive behavior. You may also need to establish a point system that involves having the child earn points that can be redeemed for a larger reward at the end of a designated period of time. For example, the child might earn points throughout the day for remembering specific behaviors (e.g., not yelling downstairs, not yelling for the dog, coming into the room to talk). If a certain number of points are earned throughout the week, the child might receive a reinforcement at the end of the week (e.g., special time with a parent, a video rental). Any behavioral modification program such as this must be worked out in advance with the parents' full cooperation.

For some children, you may also have to use a "big prize." The parents will have to agree on what the prize will be and agree to provide the prize. The child must understand that she will not get the prize unless all goals are met. If the child has a laryngeal pathology (e.g., vocal nodules), you may wait until the pathology is gone before awarding the big prize (Johnson 1985). In all fairness, be sure from the beginning that eliminating the pathology is a reasonable expectation. The reinforcement system described in the chart on the next two pages can be used with a point system.

Using a Reinforcement System

For Immediate Reinforcement of Behaviors	
Talk with the child to decide what kind of reinforcements are of interest to the child.	Any adult who is around the child throughout the day can award immediate reinforcements to the child. This might include parents, teachers, coaches, etc. Some of these reinforcements can be accumulated and turned in at the end of a specified period of time (a day, a week) to earn a bigger reward. • Stickers • Pennies • Strips of colorful paper • Post-it notes with reinforcing words written on them (e.g., "good voice," "quiet talking") • Key tags that can be purchased at office supply stores. You can write words or draw pictures. The child can carry a key ring and may enjoy putting these on the ring throughout the day. Don't forget how effective verbal praise from an adult can be. A simple "nice voice" from the teacher can be effective.
Decide if behavior charts will be used. If so, explain them to the child.	Desired behavior chart(s) can be kept in several places such as the home, the classroom, taken to the playground by the teacher or classroom aide, and/or at sports practice. The adult in that environment reminds the child that she/he will be charting during a specified period of time (e.g., "I'll be marking on your voice chart during dinner" or "I'll be marking on your voice chart during gym class.") The adult then assumes responsibility for marking either target behaviors or undesirable behaviors. An example is provided in Chapter 6, Appendix 6B, page 94.

Using Immediate or Long-Term Reinforcements

Establish with the child and the parent what long-term reinforcement (or "big prize") will be given.	The parents must play an integral role in helping to determine what the long-term reinforcement ("big prize") will be, and ideally should be responsible for providing it. It doesn't have to be an expensive prize, but if the parents are involved in selecting and providing the prize, they may be more vested in helping the child change behaviors in order to earn the prize. Depending on the age of the child, some ideas for a "big prize" include: • Going out for breakfast with one of the parents on the weekend with no siblings along • Staying up a half hour later on a school night • More computer time • A new computer game or music CD • A trip with a parent to a favorite destination (e.g., pet store, library)
Explain the chart to the child, showing how points will be recorded. 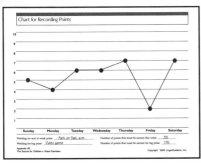	A chart for recording points earned can be kept by the SLP, or ideally, by the parent. The chart should display what prize the child is trying to earn. (See example to the left.) The chart allows the adult to record the number of points earned during the specified period of time. A blank form is provided in Appendix 4B, page 55, to record points.

Gaining the support of the parents and other adults

With most voice disorders in children, it is necessary to have the full support and participation of any adults the child interacts with. The child will need to make changes in the use of the vocal mechanism and will need help from the adults to monitor those changes. The adults may have to make modifications in how they interact with the child. For example, you may ask the soccer coach not to ask the child a question in practice that requires that the child shout the answer across the field. You may ask the parents to put a bell at the top of the stairs for the child to use to gain their attention. You may ask the teacher to monitor the child's voice use on the playground. It is important that each of these adults understands the child's voice problem and the plan to improve the voice.

Any psychodynamic/interpersonal issues that the child may present with will need to be discussed with the parents. If the problems are so significant that you think they will preclude successful voice therapy, you should have a discussion with the parents regarding additional intervention. For example, if the child is very aggressive and angry to the extent she can't learn to relax muscles or use an easy voice, she may need to be evaluated by a psychologist or counselor.

The child's parents will also be integral in helping to monitor changes in the child's voice. They will be with the child in a variety of situations and can record information about the child's vocal behaviors. You may ask the parents to graph or display the child's progress toward the goal. This record may be something as simple as a chart for stars on the refrigerator or something as elaborate as a graph recording number of times a vocal behavior occurs. Chapter 6 (pages 83-100) provides detailed information about changing behaviors and gives examples of charts and graphs for this purpose.

Managing Related Medical Problems

If the child has medical problems that are causing or exacerbating the voice disorder, management is critical. You may have to meet with the parents to discuss how the medical problem(s) are being managed. The short-term goal related to this (Medical Management = MM) may be selected along with any of the other goals. (See Appendix 4D, pages 57-61, for a master list of goals.) You should share your treatment plan with any physicians treating the child. Sometimes you may need to talk directly with these physicians to discuss the accompanying medical problems.

Short-term Goal:

Child will have appropriate medical management of related conditions. (MM)

Treatment Objectives:

1. Child will be seen for medical management of GERD. (MM-1)

2. Child will be seen for medical management of asthma. (MM-2)
    a. Child will use extenders on inhalers. (MM-2a)
    b. Child will rinse, gargle, and spit after use of inhalers. (MM-2b)

3. Child will be seen for medical management of allergies. (MM-3)

Though your role as SLP is not to manage medical problems, you can work closely with the physician to help the child and family implement medical recommendations. It is likely that you see the child much more frequently than the physician. This provides you the opportunity to ask the child and her parents about compliance with any medical treatments. In the case of GERD, you may be the one to provide most of the counseling and education about behavioral management of GERD. Use Appendix 4C, page 56, as a handout to teach the child and family about managing GERD.

Determining Prognosis and Length of Treatment

If, despite your best efforts, the child is not motivated to change behaviors, hold a conference with the parents. Perhaps this is not the best time to address the problem. If you decide to initiate trial therapy to see if you can help the child change her mind, the parents should be fully aware that prognosis for improvement is guarded as long as the child is not vested in the process. Perhaps there may be some aspects of the intervention that can be implemented without the child's full cooperation. For example, the parents could stop responding to the child yelling from upstairs and insist that she come into the room to talk to them and the gym teacher could involve the child in games where no yelling is allowed. Some of these partial changes may have some impact on the quality of the voice. In addition, if there are significant psychodynamic issues that have not been addressed (e.g., the child is acting out at home and using her voice to get attention), voice therapy may not be successful.

If voice therapy is to be successful, it should not be a long and drawn-out process. If a child implements the changes, an improvement in the physiology of the vocal mechanism (e.g., elimination of nodules or swelling) should take place within a six- to eight-week period of time. A short period of continued therapy may be necessary to ensure transfer of newly-learned behaviors to all settings.

Insurance/Reimbursement

Although insurance companies seem to be paying for therapy for fewer and fewer types of disorders, many still reimburse for voice therapy that is clearly related to a medical problem. It is helpful if you can provide the insurance company with a specific ICD-9 CM code or codes to describe the voice disorder when requesting preauthorization for treatment. A code to describe the hoarse vocal quality (784.49) should be accompanied by a code to describe a specific physiologic problem with the vocal mechanism if one is known. For example, if the hoarseness is due to the presence of vocal nodules, you might code 784.49 secondary to 478.5. A list of common ICD-9 CM codes is provided in Chapter 2, Appendix 2G, page 34.

Developing a Treatment Plan/IEP

The treatment plan development should be a collaborative effort between you, the child, and the child's parents. Everyone needs to agree on the goals and on the length of time estimated to reach those goals. The specific steps that will be taken toward reaching those goals and treatment techniques that will be used should be fully understood by all.

Selecting long-term goals

The first step in establishing a treatment plan is to select a long-term goal or goals. This goal should reflect where you think the child will be at the end of the intervention period. You may select more than one long-term goal, depending on the child's presenting problems.

- Child will be able to use voice in all situations without experiencing voice loss, phonation breaks, and/or pitch breaks.
- Child will present with a vocal quality that does not sound different from peers.
- Child will use adequate balance of oral and nasal resonance in all speaking tasks. (*Note: Although resonance is one of several misuse short-term goals, it might also be the only long-term goal and thus is listed here.*)

Selecting short-term goals

Short-term goals are the steps that need to be taken in order to reach the long-term goal(s). You may select multiple short-term goals, as a multi-pronged approach is often indicated. For example, you may need to help one child eliminate vocally abusive behaviors as well as adopt vocal hygiene techniques. Another child may need those goals as well as a goal to learn how to use appropriate volume. Still another child may not have any vocally abusive behaviors but may be speaking at a pitch that is inappropriate. Any of these children might have related medical conditions that need management. The goal for hyperfunction will likely be paired with the goals for reducing abuse and improving vocal hygiene. The child with a hyperfunctional vocal pattern may also need more in-depth work on a specific area of misuse (e.g., respiration, pitch) so you will need to choose some of those goals as well.

Child will have appropriate medical management of related conditions.	MM
Child will eliminate hyperfunctional use of the vocal mechanism.	HF
Child will eliminate abusive vocal behaviors.	VA
Child will adopt good vocal hygiene techniques.	VH
Child will eliminate misuse of respiration and will use adequate respiratory support.	MU-R
Child will eliminate misuse of phonation characterized by inappropriate volume and will use loudness appropriate to the situation.	MU-P-V
Child will eliminate misuse of phonation characterized by inappropriate pitch and will use optimal pitch in all situations.	MU-P-P
Child will eliminate misuse of phonation characterized by inappropriate onset and will exhibit appropriate vocal quality/easy onset.	MU-P-O
Child will eliminate misuse of resonance and will use appropriate oral and nasal resonance in a variety of speaking situations.	MU-ONR
Child will eliminate misuse of resonance and instead will focus phonation/tone appropriately within the mouth and nose area.	MU-TFR

Selecting treatment objectives

To document progress during each session, a smaller step than the short-term goal is needed. The goal must be broken into smaller steps called *treatment objectives*. Treatment objectives can be written so that they are measurable within a session. Each treatment objective provided (see Appendix 4D, pages 57-61) can be modified to include a variety of information. For example:

- percentage of time the behavior will occur
- number of times you expect that response from the child

- level of accuracy correct discrimination will occur
- situations in which you expect the behavior to occur

Because the treatment plan should be customized to the child, the treatment objectives in the appendix do not contain percentages, etc. Make these additions to the treatment objectives you choose for each child.

Including specific techniques on the treatment plan

You may want to include specific treatment techniques on the treatment plan. For example, you might teach the child *yawn-sigh* as a way for her to achieve appropriate onset. In that case, you could reword the treatment objective accordingly.

> *Example*: The child will use *yawn-sigh* to produce easy onset in words/phrases.

Developing the treatment plan

The treatment plan should contain the following information:

- identifying information about the child
- date of onset of the problem
- date of onset of treatment
- frequency and duration of sessions
- estimated length of treatment
- prognosis and what the prognosis is for (e.g., Are you making a prognosis about the child achieving "normal" vocal quality, or about the child achieving a voice that is functional for communication?)
- long-term goal(s)
- short-term goal(s)
- treatment objectives
- how progress will be monitored

Documenting Progress During Therapy

Documenting progress in therapy notes

In a medical setting (where a third party payer has authorized a limited number of therapy visits), documenting progress in each therapy note is especially important. You may be requested to send copies of those therapy notes along with any request for more visits. Utilizing a S.O.A.P. format will facilitate your documentation of both subjective and objective information. Under the objective part of the note you should record how well the child is doing on each of the assigned treatment objectives. Use the analysis part of the note to summarize how well the child is moving toward the long-term goals. Be specific in the plan part of the note to indicate not only what the child should work on before the next session, but what you plan to do with the child in the next therapy session.

S.O.A.P Notes

The well-recognized S.O.A.P. note format can be helpful because it forces you to analyze a client's performance. S.O.A.P. stands for S = Subjective, O = Objective, A = Analysis, P = Plan.

S = Subjective: Include initial observations of the client as you enter the room or anything the family has said about how the client is doing. You might include statements like "Rachel was talking loudly to her mom when I arrived," or "The mother reports that 'Rachel has remembered to use her bell to alert me to come upstairs.' "

O = Objective: Include any objective data you took in the session on your treatment objectives like percentages and client's response to your analysis and feedback. You might also reference any behavior recording charts that were turned in. You could summarize the chart, or simply state "See attached chart."

A = Analysis: Summarize and put in functional terms exactly what happened during each session. Instead of concentrating directly on the treatment objectives, talk about how progress on the treatment objectives moved the client closer toward achieving the functional goals. Use comparative statements like "better than the session yesterday" or "increased performance on percent of ability to perform exercises."

P = Plan: Explain what you intend to do in the next session. It can be as simple as "Continue per treatment plan" or can have specific suggestions. You may have noted in the session that the client does better with a new compensatory technique than you had initially determined. In this case, your plan might be to include this compensatory technique in future sessions. You might also include specific things the child has been asked to focus on between now and the next session.

Using the subsequent chapters

Since most voice problems involve hyperfunction, the treatment chapters begin with a discussion of hyperfunction. Chapter 5 (pages 70-82) describes hyperfunctional voice problems and some comprehensive approaches to address the physiological aspects of hyperfunction (Goal HF). Many of those approaches incorporate work on respiration, phonation, and resonation/focus.

Chapter 6 (pages 83-100) describes specific strategies for helping the child reduce vocal abuses and learn good vocal hygiene techniques (Goals VA & VH) in order to treat the behavioral aspects of hyperfunction. If the child has vocal abuses *and* excess tension for speaking voice (hyperfunctional voice or muscle tension dysphonia), you will need to use strategies from Chapter 5 and Chapter 6 to treat both the physiological and behavioral components of the hyperfunctional voice disorder. You would probably begin with treatment of the behavioral components by eliminating abuses and substituting more appropriate behaviors. After a few sessions, add in the comprehensive approach to treat the physiological components. Of course, if there are related medical problems, these must be addressed as well (Goal MM). See diagram A in Appendix 4E, page 62.

If you think the child has specific problem areas (e.g., phonation/volume, oral-nasal resonance) that will need more focus than provided in the hyperfunctional goals, identify these areas and select appropriate goals and treatment objectives from Chapter 7 (pages 101-102), Chapter 8 (pages 116-117), and Chapter 9 (pages 138 and 139). (See also page 50 in this chapter for a list of specific short-term goals.) By the third or fourth session, you can begin working on these activities along with the vocal abuse reduction program and the comprehensive approach. For example, if the child has significant difficulty with tension in respiration, you would add strategies and techniques from Chapter 7 (pages 101-115). See diagram B in Appendix 4E, page 62. Diagrams A and B represent the most likely treatment sequences for a child with a hyperfunctional voice.

You may encounter a child who has a hyperfunctional speaking pattern without other abuses that need to be changed. If that is the case, Chapter 5 alone, or more likely Chapter 6 with additional strategies from Chapters 7-9, could be used. You would start with the comprehensive approach and add other strategies and techniques as needed. See diagram C in Appendix 4E, page 63.

If the child has vocal abuse but not a hyperfunctional vocal pattern for speech, you can use Chapter 6 and that might be all you need. However, if you note particular problem areas, you might also use information from Chapters 7-9 to target specific problem areas. For example, if the child talks loudly all the time, you might draw additional strategies from Chapter 8 (pages 116-136). See diagram D in Appendix 4E, page 63.

Summary

To help make planning and implementing therapy more efficient, additional appendices for this chapter include:

- Appendix 4F (page 64): *Treatment Plan and Discharge Summary*—You can use this as a template or as an example to design your own form.

- Appendix 4G.1 (page 65): *Sample Treatment Plan for Vocal Abuse With Vocal Hygiene*—This example shows how goals and treatment objectives might be written for a child who needs to eliminate vocal abuse and improve vocal hygiene. There are no related medical problems and no additional work is needed on problem areas. The D treatment sequence on page 63 (without addressing the dotted line areas) would reflect the treatment for such a child.

- Appendix 4G.2 (page 66): This is the same as the treatment plan in 4G.1, but it is a more detailed treatment plan for vocal abuse with vocal hygiene. This one shows how you can include more specific information such as abusive behaviors, alternative behaviors, who is monitoring the child, etc.

- Appendix 4G.3 (page 67): *Sample Discharge Summary for Vocal Abuse With Vocal Hygiene* (Note: When the plan is established, use the right-hand column to indicate how you will monitor progress. Once the treatment plan becomes a discharge summary, replace the monitoring information with discharge status.)

- Appendix 4H (page 68): *Sample Treatment Plan for Vocal Misuse*—This plan is for child who is misusing her voice in the areas of volume and onset and also has related medical problems that need to be managed.

- Appendix 4I (page 69): *Sample Treatment Plan for Vocal Hyperfunction*—This sample uses parts of the comprehensive approach to treating hyperfunction with one vocal hygiene goal added. This would be similar to the treatment sequence C on page 63. The optional areas (represented by dotted lines) are not being addressed with this child.

Respiratory, Phonatory, and Resonance Systems

Lungs with larynx, front view	Inside larynx – normal
Side view lungs, larynx, and nasopharynx	**Inside larynx – nodules**

Chart for Recording Points

Sunday	Monday	Tuesday	Wednesday	Thursday	Friday	Saturday

10

9

8

7

6

5

4

3

2

1

End-of-week prize: _____

Big prize: _____

Number of points that must be earned this week: _____

Number of points that must be earned for big prize: _____

Appendix 4B
The Source for Children's Voice Disorders

Reducing Reflux

To help reduce reflux, have your child:

1. Always eat in a relaxed, calm setting.

2. Eat smaller meals throughout the day rather than three large meals. If the stomach is over-full, reflux is more likely.

3. Always include some protein foods (lean meat or poultry, cottage cheese, or very low-fat cheese) in each meal. Keep fat content of meals low.

4. Try separating fluid and solid food intake. Some children have fewer symptoms if they eat the entire meal and then drink.

5. Avoid late evening meals or snacks. This also applies to drinking a glass of water or taking pills before bed.

6. Wait for at least an hour to lie down after having anything to eat or drink.

7. Sleep on a bed that has the head elevated about six inches. This is best done with blocks under the legs of the head of the bed. It is not effective to add extra pillows as this just elevates the head and shoulders.

8. Lose weight if he or she is overweight. Discuss a sensible weight-reduction plan with your child's pediatrician.

9. Avoid tight clothing around the waistline. This puts pressure on the sphincter at the top of the stomach that is supposed to keep the stomach contents from re-entering the esophagus.

10. Avoid bending over. Instead, your child should stoop down and keep his/her back straight.

11. Avoid lifting heavy objects.

12. Some foods make reflux worse, but this varies from person to person. The following is a list of potential irritants. Help your child analyze which foods cause the symptoms of reflux to increase.

- caffeine (coffee, tea, cola, chocolate, cocoa)
- mint
- peppers
- carbonated beverages
- citrus (oranges, grapefruits)

- chili powder and other spices
- tomatoes and tomato products
- cured and "spiced" meats (lunchmeat, sausage, hot dogs)
- pickled items

Master List of Long-term Goals, Short-term Goals, and Treatment Objectives

Long-term Goals

- Child will be able to use voice in all situations without experiencing voice loss, phonation breaks, and/or pitch breaks.
- Child will present with a vocal quality that does not sound different from peers.
- Child will use adequate balance of oral and nasal resonance in all speaking tasks. (*Note: Although resonance is one of several misuse short-term goals, it might also be the only long-term goal and thus is listed here.*)

Short-term Goal for Medical Management (STG-MM)

Child will have appropriate medical management of related conditions. (MM)

Treatment Objectives

1. Child will be seen for medical management of GERD. (MM-1)

2. Child will be seen for medical management of asthma. (MM-2)

   a. Child will use extenders on inhalers. (MM-2a)

   b. Child will rinse, gargle, and spit after use of inhalers. (MM-2b)

3. Child will be seen for medical management of allergies. (MM-3)

Short-term Goal for Hyperfunctional Use of the Vocal Mechanism (STG-HF)

Child will eliminate the hyperfunctional use of the vocal mechanism. (HF)

Treatment Objectives

1. Child will discriminate between tense, hyperfunctional phonation and appropriate phonation as modeled by SLP. (HF-1)

2. Child will identify location of muscle tension. (HF-2)

   a. phonatory muscles (HF-2a)

   b. oro-pharyngeal muscles (HF-2b)

   c. respiratory muscles (HF-2c)

3. Child will use techniques to reduce muscle tension in: (HF-3)

   a. phonatory muscles (HF-3a)

   b. oro-pharyngeal musculature (HF-3b)

   c. respiratory muscles (HF-3c)

4. Child will utilize techniques to eliminate muscle tension during: (HF-4)
   a. words and phrases (HF-4a)
   b. sentence level utterances (HF-4b)
   c. conversation (HF-4c)

Short-term Goal for Vocal Abuse (STG-VA)

Child will eliminate abusive vocal behaviors. (VA)

Treatment Objectives

1. Child will identify vocally abusive behaviors. (VA-1)
2. Child will collect reliable baseline data on abusive behaviors. (VA-2)
3. Child will identify acceptable alternatives to vocally abusive behaviors. (VA-3)
4. Child will reduce/eliminate the following abusive behaviors: _____. (VA-4)
5. Child will substitute acceptable alternatives to vocally abusive behaviors. (VA-5)

Short-term Goal for Vocal Hygiene (STG-VH)

Child will adopt good vocal hygiene techniques. (VH)

Treatment Objectives

1. Child will drink water to keep vocal mechanism hydrated. (VH-1)
2. Child will get an adequate amount of sleep. (VH-2)
3. Child will avoid beverages and food with caffeine. (VH-3)
4. Child will avoid exposure to smoke/chemicals. (VH-4)
5. Child will use an acceptable volume. (VH-5)
6. Child will speak to others from an appropriate distance. (VH-6)

Short-term Goals for Misuse

(Note: Some of these may be appropriate additional goals/treatment objectives for the child with vocal hyperfunction. First see goal HF and the treatment objectives to determine if they adequately describe what the child needs to address.)

Short-term Goal for Misuse of Respiration (STG-MU-R)

Child will eliminate misuse of respiration and will use adequate respiratory support. (MU-R)

Treatment Objectives

1. Child will demonstrate understanding of difference in diaphragmatic and clavicular (or other abnormal patterns) breathing. (MU-R-1)
   a. when modeled by SLP (MU-R-1a)
   b. when the child imitates the patterns (MU-R-1b)

2. Child will use diaphragmatic breathing in supine on: (MU-R-2)
    a. simple exhalations (MU-R-2a)
    b. production of vowel sounds (MU-R-2b)
    c. imitation of phrases and sentences (MU-R-2c)

3. Child will use diaphragmatic breathing when standing on: (MU-R-3)
    a. simple exhalations (MU-R-3a)
    b. production of vowel sounds (MU-R-3b)
    c. imitation of phrases and sentences (MU-R-3c)

4. Child will use diaphragmatic breathing when sitting on: (MU-R-4)
    a. simple exhalations (MU-R-4a)
    b. production of vowel sounds (MU-R-4b)
    c. imitation of phrases and sentences (MU-R-4c)

5. Child will remember to take an adequate breath before beginning to speak in: (MU-R-5)
    a. short answers (MU-R-5a)
    b. reading passages (MU-R-5b)
    c. monologues (MU-R-5c)
    d. conversations (MU-R-5d)

6. Child will avoid speaking on low air by pausing for a breath during: (MU-R-6)
    a. reading passages (MU-R-6a)
    b. monologues (MU-R-6b)
    c. conversations (MU-R-6c)

Short-term Goal for Misuse of Phonation Characterized by Inappropriate Volume (STG-MU-P-V)

Child will eliminate misuse of phonation characterized by inappropriate volume and will use loudness appropriate to the situation. (MU-P-V)

Treatment Objectives

1. Child will discriminate between three vocal loudness levels modeled by SLP. (MU-P-V-1)

2. Child will produce each of the three loudness levels in: (MU-P-V-2)
    a. words and short phrases (MU-P-V-2a)
    b. sentences (MU-P-V-2b)
    c. conversation (MU-P-V-2c)

3. Child will select and use appropriate loudness level in a variety of situations. (MU-P-V-3)

59

Short-term Goal for Misuse of Phonation Characterized by Inappropriate Pitch (STG-MU-P-P)

Child will eliminate misuse of phonation characterized by inappropriate pitch and will use optimal pitch in all situations. (MU-P-P)

Treatment Objectives

1. Child will discriminate between low and high pitches modeled by SLP. (MU-P-P-1)

2. Child will discriminate between inappropriate and target pitch in audiotape/live samples of own speech. (MU-P-P-2)

3. Child will consistently use target pitch (optimal fundamental frequency) in: (MU-P-P-3)
   a. words and short phrases (MU-P-P-3a)
   b. sentences (MU-P-P-3b)
   c. conversation (MU-P-P-3c)

Short-term Goal for Misuse of Phonation Characterized by Inappropriate Onset (STG-MU-P-O)

Child will eliminate misuse of phonation characterized by inappropriate onset and will exhibit appropriate vocal quality/easy onset. (MU-P-O)

Treatment Objectives

1. Child will discriminate between breathy, hard attack and adequate onset of phonation modeled by SLP. (MU-P-O-1)

2. Child will discriminate between breathy, hard attack and adequate onset in audiotape/live samples of own phonation. (MU-P-O-2)

3. Child will produce appropriate/easy onset on/in: (MU-P-O-3)
   a. vowels (MU-P-O-3a)
   b. vowel-initiated words and phrases (MU-P-O-3b)
   c. words and phrases starting with consonants (MU-P-O-3c)
   d. sentences (MU-P-O-3d)
   e. conversation (MU-P-O-3e)

Short-term Goal for Misuse of Resonance/Use of Appropriate Oral and Nasal Resonance (STG-MU-ONR)

Child will eliminate misuse of resonance and will use appropriate oral and nasal resonance in a variety of speaking situations. (MU-ONR)

Treatment Objectives

1. Child will discriminate oral vs. hypernasal resonance as modeled by SLP. (MU-ONR-1)

2. Child will discriminate between oral and nasal resonance in audiotape/live samples of own speech. (MU-ONR-2)

3. Child will reduce perceived hypernasality on/in: (MU-ONR-3)

    a. vowels (MU-ONR-3a)

    b. words (MU-ONR-3b)

    c. phrases and sentences (MU-ONR-3c)

    d. conversation (MU-ONR-3d)

Short-term Goal for Misuse of Tone Focus/Resonance (STG-MU-TFR)

Child will eliminate misuse of resonance and instead will focus the phonation/tone appropriately within the mouth and nose area. (MU-TFR)

Treatment Objectives

1. Child will discriminate between thin (forward focus), muffled (cul-de-sac) resonance and appropriately balanced oral resonance when modeled by SLP. (MU-TFR-1)

2. Child will discriminate between thin (forward focus), muffled (cul-de-sac) resonance and appropriately balanced oral resonance in audiotape/live samples of own speech. (MU-TFR-2)

3. Child will utilize resonance that is balanced between the front and back of the mouth on/in: (MU-TFR-3)

    a. vowels (MU-TFR-3a)

    b. words (MU-TFR-3b)

    c. phrases and sentences (MU-TFR-3c)

    d. conversation (MU-TFR-3d)

4. Child will discriminate between phonation/tone focused in the throat and that focused in the mouth and nose area when modeled by SLP. (MU-TFR-4)

5. Child will discriminate between phonation/tone focused in the throat and that focused in the mouth and nose area in audiotape/live samples of own speech. (MU-TFR-5)

6. Child will utilize resonance that is appropriately focused in the mouth and nose area on/in: (MU-TFR-6)

    a. vowels (MU-TFR-6a)

    b. words (MU-TFR-6b)

    c. phrases and sentences (MU-TFR-6c)

    d. conversation (MU-TFR-6d)

Sample Treatment Sequences for Vocal Problems*

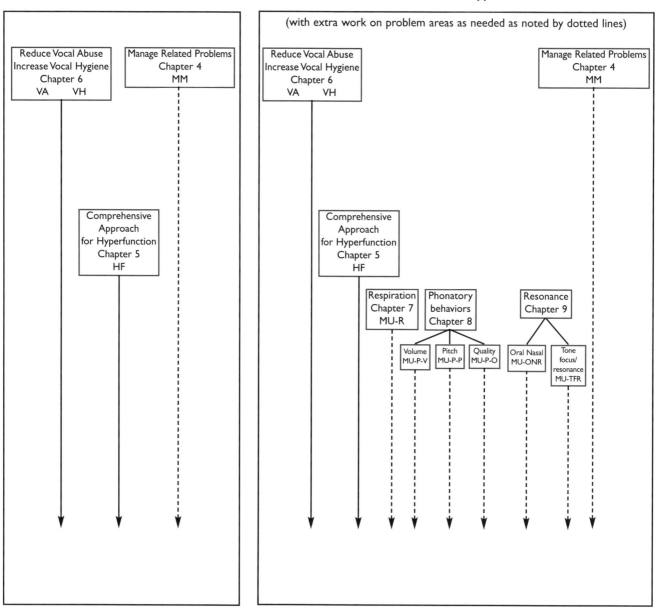

A

Vocal Abuse with Hyperfunction

B

Vocal Abuse with Hyperfunction

(with extra work on problem areas as needed as noted by dotted lines)

Reduce Vocal Abuse
Increase Vocal Hygiene
Chapter 6
VA   VH

Manage Related Problems
Chapter 4
MM

Comprehensive
Approach
for Hyperfunction
Chapter 5
HF

Respiration
Chapter 7
MU-R

Phonatory
behaviors
Chapter 8

Volume
MU-P-V

Pitch
MU-P-P

Quality
MU-P-O

Resonance
Chapter 9

Oral Nasal
MU-ONR

Tone
focus/
resonance
MU-TFR

* If there are accompanying medical problems, management is essential and thus is included in each sample treatment sequence.

C

Hyperfunction Without Abuse

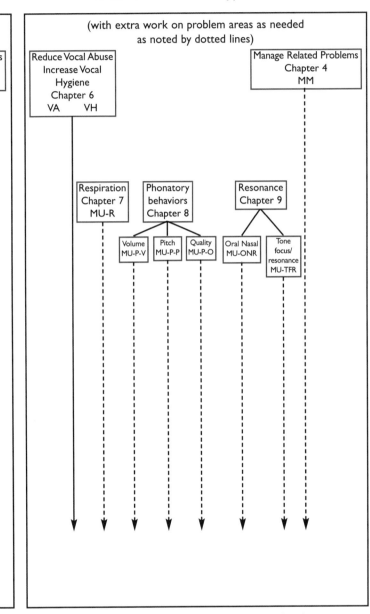

(with extra work on problem areas as needed as noted by dotted lines)

Comprehensive Approach for Hyperfunction
Chapter 5
HF

Manage Related Problems
Chapter 4
MM

Respiration
Chapter 7
MU-R

Phonatory behaviors
Chapter 8

Volume
MU-P-V

Pitch
MU-P-P

Quality
MU-P-O

Resonance
Chapter 9

Oral Nasal
MU-ONR

Tone focus/ resonance
MU-TFR

(See page 69 for sample of treatment plan.)

D

Vocal Abuse Without Hyperfunction

(with extra work on problem areas as needed as noted by dotted lines)

Reduce Vocal Abuse
Increase Vocal Hygiene
Chapter 6
VA   VH

Manage Related Problems
Chapter 4
MM

Respiration
Chapter 7
MU-R

Phonatory behaviors
Chapter 8

Volume
MU-P-V

Pitch
MU-P-P

Quality
MU-P-O

Resonance
Chapter 9

Oral Nasal
MU-ONR

Tone focus/ resonance
MU-TFR

(See pages 65-67 for sample treatment plans.)

Treatment Plan and Discharge Summary

Client's Name _____   Birthdate _____   Age _____

Date therapy initiated _____   Date therapy terminated _____

Frequency and duration of treatment sessions _____

Total Units _____

Therapy conducted at _____

Onset date of current problem _____

Diagnosis _____

Prognosis _____

Estimated length of treatment _____

Follow-up _____

Long-term goals _____

_____

Short-term Goals/Treatment Objectives	How Progress Will Be Monitored/ Discharge Status

Summary Statement _____

_____

_____

_____

_____

_____
Speech-Language Pathologist

Sample Treatment Plan for Vocal Abuse With Vocal Hygiene (generic)

Client's Name ___Ned Nodules___ Birthdate ___1-8-97___ Age ___8-1___

Date therapy initiated ___2-14-05___ Date therapy terminated _____

Frequency and duration of treatment sessions ___1x week; half-hour___

Total Units _____

Therapy conducted at ___Very Good Voice Clinic___

Onset date of current problem ___11-04___

Diagnosis ___Small bilateral vocal nodules with some laryngeal edema — hoarseness___

Prognosis ___Excellent for eliminating nodules and achieving adequate vocal quality___

Estimated length of treatment ___10-12 weeks___

Follow-up _____

Long-term Goals ___1. Child will be able to use voice in all situations without experiencing voice loss.___

___2. Child will present with a vocal quality that does not sound different than peers.___

Short-term Goals/Treatment Objectives	How Progress Will Be Monitored/ Discharge Status
Child will eliminate abusive vocal behaviors. (VA) 1. Child will identify vocally abusive behaviors. (VA-1) 2. Child will collect reliable baseline data on these abusive behaviors. (VA-2) 3. Child will identify acceptable alternatives to vocally abusive behaviors. (VA-3) 4. Child will reduce/eliminate abusive patterns. (VA-4) 5. Child will substitute acceptable alternatives to vocally abusive behaviors. (VA-5) Child will adopt good vocal hygiene techniques. (VH) 6. Child will drink water to keep vocal mechanism hydrated. (VH-1)	VA 1. SLP will work with child to identify behaviors. 2. Homeroom teacher, coach, and gym teacher as well as parents will help child collect data. 3. SLP and child will complete the *Things I Can Do Instead That Won't Hurt My Voice* form. 4. Parents and teachers will help child monitor and collect data concerning abusive patterns on *Chart to Record Behaviors to Reduce and Substitute* and this will be turned in weekly to SLP to graph. 5. Parents and teachers will help child monitor and collect data on acceptable alternatives on *Chart to Record Behaviors to Reduce and Substitute* and this will be turned in weekly to the SLP to graph. VH 6. Teacher will monitor that child gets drink in hall on way to gym class and after lunch. Parents will monitor amount of water drunk from bottle she'll carry at home.

Sample Treatment Plan for Vocal Abuse With Vocal Hygiene (detailed)

Client's Name ___Ned Nodules___ Birthdate ___1-8-97___ Age ___8-1___

Date therapy initiated ___2-14-05___ Date therapy terminated _____

Frequency and duration of treatment sessions ___1x week; half-hour___

Total Units _____

Therapy conducted at ___Very Good Voice Clinic___

Onset date of current problem ___11-04___

Diagnosis ___Small bilateral vocal nodules with some laryngeal edema — hoarseness___

Prognosis ___Excellent for eliminating nodules and achieving adequate vocal quality___

Estimated length of treatment ___10-12 weeks___

Follow-up _____

Long-term Goals ___1. Child will be able to use voice in all situations without experiencing voice loss.___

___2. Child will present with a vocal quality that does not sound different than peers.___

Short-term Goals/Treatment Objectives	How Progress Will Be Monitored/ Discharge Status

Child will eliminate abusive vocal behaviors. (VA)
1. Child will identify vocally abusive behaviors. (VA-1)
2. Child will collect reliable baseline data on these abusive behaviors: (VA-2)
  a. Yelling on playground
  b. Screaming at sister at home
  c. Making funny noises
  d. Not taking turns in conversation
3. Child will identify acceptable alternatives to vocally abusive behaviors. (VA-3)
4. Child will reduce/eliminate abusive patterns: (VA-4)
  a. Yelling on playground
  b. Screaming at sister at home
  c. Making funny noises
  d. Not taking turns in conversation
5. Child will substitute acceptable alternatives to vocally abusive behaviors. (VA-5)
  a. Clapping hands or whistling for attention
  b. Using an angry face when mad at sister
  c. Use of funny noises will be eliminated
  d. Making sure the other person gets equal number of turns
Child will adopt good vocal hygiene techniques. (VH)
6. Child will drink water to keep vocal mechanism hydrated. (VH-1)
	VA
	1. SLP will work with child to identify behaviors.
	2. Homeroom teacher, coach, and gym teacher as well as parents will help child collect data.
	3. SLP and child will complete the *Things I Can Do Instead That Won't Hurt My Voice* form.
	4. Parents and teachers will help child monitor and collect data concerning abusive patterns on *Chart to Record Behaviors to Reduce and Substitute* and this will be turned in weekly to SLP to graph.
	  a. Teacher
	  b. Parents
	  c. Parents and after-school care
	  d. Parents and teachers
	5. Parents and teachers will help child monitor and collect data on acceptable alternatives on *Chart to Record Behaviors to Reduce and Substitute* and this will be turned in weekly to the SLP to graph.
	VH
	6. Teacher will monitor that child gets drink in hall on way to gym class and after lunch. Parents will monitor amount of water drunk from bottle she'll carry at home.

Sample Discharge Summary for Vocal Abuse With Vocal Hygiene

Client's Name __Ned Nodules__   Birthdate __1-8-97__   Age __8-1__

Date therapy initiated __2-14-05__   Date therapy terminated __5-16-05__

Frequency and duration of treatment sessions __1x week; half-hour__

Total Units __22 units__

Therapy conducted at __Very Good Voice Clinic__

Onset date of current problem __11-04__

Diagnosis __Small bilateral vocal nodules with some laryngeal edema — hoarseness__

Prognosis __Excellent for eliminating nodules and achieving adequate vocal quality__

Estimated length of treatment __10-12 weeks__

Follow-up __Call client's parents in one month__

Long-term Goals __1. Child will be able to use voice in all situations without experiencing voice loss.__

__2. Child will present with a vocal quality that does not sound different than peers.__

Short-term Goals/Treatment Objectives	How Progress Will Be Monitored/ Discharge Status

Child will eliminate abusive vocal behaviors. (VA)
1. Child will identify vocally abusive behaviors. (VA-1)
2. Child will collect reliable baseline data on these abusive behaviors: (VA-2)
   a. Yelling on playground
   b. Screaming at sister at home
   c. Making funny noises
   d. Not taking turns in conversation
3. Child will identify acceptable alternatives to vocally abusive behaviors. (VA-3)
4. Child will reduce/eliminate abusive patterns: (VA-4)
   a. Yelling on playground
   b. Screaming at sister at home
   c. Making funny noises
   d. Not taking turns in conversation
5. Child will substitute acceptable alternatives to vocally abusive behaviors. (VA-5)
   a. Clapping hands or whistling for attention
   b. Using an angry face when mad at sister
   c. Use of funny noises will be eliminated
   d. Making sure the other person gets equal number of turns
 	
Child will adopt good vocal hygiene techniques. (VH)
6. Child will drink water to keep vocal mechanism hydrated. (VH-1)
	Discharge Status: VA
	1. Achieved
	2. Achieved. Baseline data counts were:
	   a. 25 times/week
	   b. 8 times/week
	   c. 10 times/day on average
	   d. in conversations monitored over 3 days, this was observed 80%
	3. Achieved
	4. Child has done a very good job at reducing these behaviors. Last measures taken indicated:
	   a. 3 times/week
	   b. 1 time/week
	   c. 2 times/day on average
	   d. Not taking turns occurs in only about 30% of the conversations monitored, and usually only in "competitive" conversations on the playground and at sports practice
	5. Child is using these behaviors very well:
	   a. Noted 6 times/week on playground
	   b. Mother reports child is consistently using the angry face
	   c. Child will not use funny noises.
	   d. Child has taken pride in applying this new turn-taking skill.
	6. Parents report bottle is empty at end of day 5/7 days. Teacher reports 100% compliance with getting drink in the hall.

Sample Treatment Plan for Vocal Misuse
(in areas of volume and onset)

Client's Name ___Hard Loud "HL" Talker___ Birthdate ___4-29-99___ Age ___6-5___

Date therapy initiated ___9-25-05___

Frequency and duration of treatment sessions ___2x week; half-hour___

Therapy conducted at ___Excellent Elementary___

Onset date of current problem ___For years___

Diagnosis ___Intermittent hoarse vocal quality; no laryngeal pathology___

Prognosis ___Good for eliminating vocal misuse___

Estimated length of treatment ___12-24 weeks___

Long-term Goals ___1. Child will present with a vocal quality that does not sound different than peers.___

Short-term Goals/Treatment Objectives	How Progress Will Be Monitored/ Discharge Status

Child will eliminate misuse of phonation characterized by inappropriate volume and use loudness appropriate to the situation. (MU-P-V)
 1. Child will discriminate between three vocal loudness levels modeled by SLP. (MU-P-V-1)
 2. Child will produce each of the three loudness levels in: (MU-P-V-2)
     a. Words and short phrases
     b. Sentence level utterances
     c. Conversation
 3. Child will select and use appropriate loudness level in a variety of situations: (MU-P-V-3)
     a. Classroom conversations
     b. Talking with sibling in back seat of car
     c. Dinner table conversations
     d. In the hall at school
     e. In the cafeteria
	1. SLP will monitor accuracy in therapy.
	
	 2. SLP will monitor in therapy.
	
	 3. Teacher will monitor in classroom, hall, and cafeteria. Parents will monitor in the car and at the dinner table. Each will dispense tokens for target volume. Tokens will be charted weekly by parents on *Chart For Recording Points*

Child will eliminate misuse of phonation characterized by inappropriate onset and exhibit appropriate vocal quality/onset. (MU-P-O)
 4. Child will discriminate between hard attack and adequate onset of phonation modeled by SLP. (MU-P-O-1)
 5. Child will discriminate between hard attack and adequate onset from audiotape/live samples of own speech. (MU-P-O-2)
 6. Child will produce easy onset on/in: (MU-P-O-3)
     a. Vowels
     b. Vowel-initiated words and phrases
     c. Words and phrases starting with consonants
     d. Sentences
     e. Conversation
	4. SLP will monitor in therapy.
	
	 5. SLP will monitor progress in therapy.
	
	 6. SLP will collect data in therapy.

Child will have appropriate medical management of related conditions. (MM)
 7. Child will be seen for medical management of asthma. (MM-1)
     a. Child will use extenders on inhalers.
     b. Child will rinse, gargle, and spit after use of inhalers.
	7. Pulmonologist will monitor progress of asthma management, but parents will monitor use of extenders on inhalers at home as well as gargling after each use of inhaler.

Sample Treatment Plan for Vocal Hyperfunction

Client's Name ___Tense Takisha___   Birthdate ___7-1-94___   Age ___10-8___

Date therapy initiated ___3-5-05___   Date therapy terminated _____

Frequency and duration of treatment sessions ___2x week___

Total Units _____

Therapy conducted at ___Perfect Private Practice___

Onset date of current problem _____

Diagnosis ___Lateral compression of supraglottal structures with phonation – hyperfunctional, hoarse harsh voice___

Prognosis ___Good for eliminating hyperfunction___

Estimated length of treatment ___3-4 months___

Follow-up _____

Long-term Goals ___1. Child will be able to use voice in all situations without experiencing voice loss and phonation breaks.___

___2. Child will present with a vocal quality that does not sound different than peers.___

Note: This plan contains some specific areas of tension that were identified during evaluation.

Short-term Goals/Treatment Objectives	How Progress Will Be Monitored/ Discharge Status

Child will eliminate the hyperfunctional use of the vocal mechanism. (HF)
1. Child will discriminate between tense, hyperfunctional phonation and appropriate phonation as modeled by the SLP. (HF-1)
2. Child will identify location of muscle tension. (HF-2)
 	
3. Child will use techniques to reduce muscle tension in: (HF-3)
   a. Phonatory muscles — yawn-sigh and front focus sounds to eliminate tension in phonatory muscles
   b. Respiratory muscles — child will use diaphragmatic breathing
4. Child will utilize front focus sounds techniques to eliminate muscle tension during: (HF-4)
   a. Words and phrases
   b. Sentence level utterances
   c. Conversation
 	
Child will adopt good vocal hygiene techniques. (VH)
5. Child will drink water to keep vocal mechanism hydrated. (VH-1)
	1. SLP will monitor accuracy in therapy.
	
	2. SLP will monitor for accuracy as determined by child's verbal responses and ability to point to area of tension.
	3. Child will use:
	   a. Yawn-sigh and front focus sounds to eliminate tension in phonatory muscles. This will be monitored by SLP.
	   b. Child will use diaphragmatic breathing to be monitored by SLP.
	
	4. Child will apply front focus sounds to different speech tasks, monitored by SLP in therapy and parents and teachers in other situations.
	
	5. Child will record # of ounces taken each day (based on the water bottle she will carry) on the chart.

5 | Treating the Hyperfunctional Voice

The vast majority of voice problems presented by children will be problems of hyperfunction. Boone et al. (2005) describe vocal hyperfunction as "the involvement of excessive muscle force and physical effort in the systems of respiration, phonation, and resonance" (p. 8). You may note the hyperfunction in the extrinsic muscles in the neck (Stemple et al. 1980, Aronson 1990), in the respiratory system (Sapienza et al. 1997), and even in the jaw and mouth.

The relationship between hyperfunction and vocal abuse

Most vocally abusive behaviors could be called hyperfunctional. Slamming the vocal folds together in a cough or throat clear certainly involves hyperfuntion of the mechanism. Talking too loudly without good breath support will undoubtedly put a strain on the vocal mechanism.

In this book, we view hyperfunction as a voice consistently produced with too much tension. Another term frequently used to describe this pattern was coined by Rammage et al. (2001): *muscle tension dysphonia*. Therefore, a child who has some vocal abuses (e.g., throat clearing, screaming on the playground) may have a hoarse vocal quality. If he doesn't use too much force and tension in his everyday speaking voice, he would not be considered to have a hyperfunctional voice. However, if he persists in the use of these abusive behaviors, he is likely to develop an organic problem (e.g., nodules, edema). This organic problem may trigger use of a hyperfunctional vocal pattern.

Chapter 6 (pages 83-100) describes specific strategies for helping the child reduce vocal abuses and learn good vocal hygiene techniques. This is considered treating the behavioral aspects of hyperfunction. Verdolini (in Hillman & Verdolini 1999) describes this as "treating the software" (i.e., making changes in the cognitive and neural programs that drive voice production). This chapter, however, provides information about more comprehensive approaches to address the physiological aspects of hyperfunction. Many of those approaches incorporate work on respiration, phonation, and resonance/focus. Verdolini calls this "treating the hardware" (i.e., making alterations in the muscle and mucosal composition through exercise).

Chapters 7 through 9 (pages 101-156) provide information and techniques for addressing each of the following components: respiration; phonation (e.g., loudness, pitch, quality/onset), and resonance. These chapters can be used to supplement the comprehensive approach to hyperfunction.

Types of Hyperfunction

Hillman (in Hillman & Verdolini 1999) describes two types of hyperfunction:

- Primary hyperfunction
- Secondary/reactive hyperfunction

Primary hyperfunction means that the hyperfunction of the vocal mechanism is the primary problem. It can cause organic changes in the vocal mechanism such as edema, nodules, or polyps. (See Chapter 1, pages 9-12). It can also cause or contribute to functional voice disorders (those with no organic pathology) such as functional dysphonia, vocal fatigue, or even aphonia.

Secondary/reactive hyperfunction means that the hyperfunction of the vocal mechanism is in reaction to (secondary to) some organic change. (See Chapter 1, pages 13-15). For example, a child with a paralyzed vocal fold might use a reactive hyperfunctional voice in order to be heard. In a more common scenario, a child might experience an upper respiratory infection with some laryngitis (hoarseness) and finds he has to push hard to produce a voice that can be heard. After the laryngitis has resolved, the child might continue to exhibit the hyperfunctional voice patterns.

Hyperfunction can result in a different sounding voice

Hillman et al. (1989) utilized a theoretical framework that describes different types of hyperfunction:

- **Adducted vocal hyperfunction**: The increased muscle tension results in over-approximation of all or parts of the vocal folds. This is called an *abnormal glottal closure pattern*. There may be stiffness in vocal fold structures. The child with adducted vocal hyperfunction would use increased subglottal pressure to produce the voice and much force when closing the vocal folds. Initially the voice might sound hoarse and strained. If the pattern persists, lesions can develop on the vocal folds. Once lesions are in place, the voice may additionally sound somewhat breathy. This is because air escapes past the lesion during phonation (like trying to close a door when someone's foot is stuck in the opening).

- **Non-adducted vocal hyperfunction**: The increased muscle tension results in under-approximation of the vocal folds. There may be stiffness in vocal fold structures. The child will use increased subglottal pressure to produce the voice. The voice will sound weak or breathy. The child may complain that talking makes him tired. You may hear a normal-sounding voice on vegetative tasks like a cough or laugh. It may seem odd that over-using the muscles would result in a voice that sounds breathy. Try whispering for a minute or two and then notice how much excess muscle tension you feel in your throat to get the idea.

How do you know if the child is using a hyperfunctional voice?

If the child has had an instrumental examination of the voice that included nasendoscopy, or preferably videostroboscopy, the report will describe the hyperfunction. Over-adduction of the false folds and arytenoids might be reported or the report might use the terms *hyperfunction* or *muscle tension dysphonia*. Using flexible and/or rigid endoscopy, the SLP or otolaryngologist would have been able to observe the use of excess muscle tension above the level of the true vocal folds. The endoscopist may give a very specific description of where the muscle tension is observed.

- The child may be using excess tension in the false (ventricular) folds, described as *lateral compression*.

- The child may exhibit excess tension that results in the arytenoids tipping so far forward they almost touch the epiglottis, called *anterior-posterior compression*.

The true vocal folds might also be approximated so tightly that it is difficult for the air to pass over the folds. This tightness might be described as:

- Over-adduction (squeezing of the arytenoids)
- Over-adduction with bulging of the vocal processes
- Posterior chink that extends into the membranous glottis; often associated with vocal nodules
- Anterior chink related to lesions
- Anterior and posterior chink; forms an hourglass configuration on closure
- Lack of closure along entire length

On a clinical examination, the child's voice could present with one of two distinct patterns:

- The child's voice might sound tight and strained in addition to sounding hoarse. The terms *strained* or *strangled* might be used to describe the voice. You might even observe excessive muscle tension in the strap muscles of the neck. The child may appear to almost be pushing the voice out (i.e., adducted vocal hyperfunction). If this pattern has resulted in the development of nodules, for example, the voice may also sound breathy.

- The child's voice may sound breathy or be described as weak (i.e., non-adducted vocal hyperfunction). This is the result of the child under-approximating the folds due to too much tension. You may hear a normal-sounding voice on vegetative tasks like a cough or laugh.

Treating Hyperfunction

Chapter 4 (pages 42-69) contains a description of how treatment for hyperfunction might be structured. It includes sample flow charts to illustrate the timing of the different aspects of treatment. This chapter will now focus on describing a comprehensive approach to treating the physiological aspects of the hyperfunction (i.e., teaching the child not to use too much muscle tension when speaking). The chapter will reference activities and techniques that are described in more detail in Chapters 7-9 (pages 101-156).

The sequence described here is an integration of ideas and techniques from four main sources:

- Resonant Voice Therapy (Lessac 1973, Verdolini 1998)
- Facilitating Approaches (Boone et al. 2005)
- Vocal Function Exercises (Stemple et al. 1994)
- Management of the Voice and Its Disorders (Rammage et al. 2001)

What these approaches have in common is reflected in the goals and treatment objectives written for treating hyperfunction. That is, the child has to be able to tell what you mean by using too much muscle tension and has to be able to discern which parts of the body involved in phonation are too tight. This might include muscles of the face, mouth, neck, and shoulders (oro-pharyngeal), the larynx (vocal folds and supraglottal structures), and the chest and stomach (respiration). Then the child has to learn how to release that muscle tension and produce a better voice. These approaches all use techniques to get the child to re-focus the resonance of the voice in the front of the face (nose and mouth) while maintaining no excess tension.

Short-term Goal

Child will eliminate the hyperfunctional use of the vocal mechanism. (HF)

Treatment Objectives

1. Child will discriminate between tense, hyperfunctional phonation and appropriate phonation as modeled by SLP. (HF-1)

2. Child will identify location of muscle tension in: (HF-2)
   a. phonatory muscles (HF-2a)
   b. oro-pharyngeal musculature (HF-2b)
   c. respiratory muscles (HF-2c)

3. Child will use techniques to reduce muscle tension in: (HF-3)
   a. phonatory muscles (HF-3a)
   b. oro-pharyngeal musculature (HF-3b)
   c. respiratory muscles (HF-3c)

4. Child will use techniques to eliminate muscle tension during: (HF-4)
   a. words and phrases (HF-4a)
   b. sentences (HF-4b)
   c. conversation (HF-4c)

Explaining hyperfunction to the child

In order for the child to be able to tell when he is using a hyperfunctional voice pattern, he has to understand what is meant by too much muscle tension. It is probably easiest to start with helping the child understand muscle tension in a more visible, easily manipulated muscle. You can have the child feel your bicep when it is relaxed and when it is lightly tensed as you bend your arm. Then demonstrate "too much" muscle tension as you squeeze your hand toward your shoulder, making the bicep bulge. Let the child try "showing his muscle" and discriminating between just enough tension to bend the arm and the excess tension needed to make the muscle bulge. Compare this to the amount of tension used when the voice is hyperfunctional.

Helping the child discriminate between tense and appropriate phonation

HF Treatment Objective 1	Child will discriminate between tense, hyperfunctional phonation and appropriate phonation as modeled by SLP.

It will be easier for the child to identify hyperfunction when he hears it in your voice or someone else's voice before being expected to determine when he is using too much tension. Model easy, relaxed phonation. Use the appropriate picture from Appendix 5A (Relaxing Ricardo or Rita, page 79) and explain to the child that when this nice easy voice is heard, Ricardo (or Rita) is not forcing. Then demonstrate what a hyperfunctional voice might sound like. (Note: Only do this for short periods of time. Don't strain your own vocal mechanism!). Use the pictures of Straining Stan or Stephanie to match the tense voice you model.

Determining where the muscle tension is occurring

	Child will identify location of muscle tension in:
HF Treatment Objective 2	a. phonatory muscles b. oro-pharyngeal musculature c. respiratory muscles

The child may be exhibiting muscle tension not only in the larynx itself, in the glottis, and/or supraglottal structures, but also in the extrinsic muscles of the larynx and those used for articulation (oro-pharyngeal musculature) and in the muscles used for respiration.

Identifying excess muscle tension in the phonatory muscles

This may be the most difficult of the three areas to explain to the child because the larynx is not visible to the child. He can't put his hands on it and feel the tension (like he may able to do with the extrinsic musculature). Use pictures and analogies to help the child understand that the vocal folds themselves may be used with too much tension and that the muscles around the vocal folds may also be too tight.

You can use your index and middle finger in a V-shape to represent the vocal folds. Have the child move your fingers open and closed. Explain that that is how the vocal folds move without too much tension. Then tense your fingers. Try to keep your fingers open as the child tries to move them in and out.

To demonstrate what you mean by tension in the muscles around the vocal folds, create a U-shape with your other hand. Lay the two fingers in the V-shape (representing the vocal folds) in the palm of the hand in the U-shape. Have the child move your fingers easily open and closed. To demonstrate the anterior and lateral compression of the supraglottal structures, squeeze your hand closed. Then ask the child to try to move your fingers. Point out how, even though the vocal folds (fingers) themselves aren't tight, when the muscles around them are tight, they can't move well.

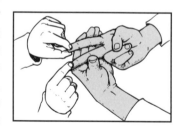

Identifying excess muscle tension in the oro-pharyngeal musculature

Muscles included in the oro-pharyngeal musculature that can become tight and affect phonation are located in the jaw, lips, tongue, front and back of the neck, and the shoulders.

All of these muscles play a role in allowing easy, relaxed phonation. If the articulators are tight, the resonance of the voice in the oral cavity will be restricted. The child may then push even harder to project the voice. Many of the muscles in the front of the neck have attachments to the larynx. Muscles in the back of the neck can become tight and rigid. When they become fixed, the muscles in the front of the neck may become fixed as well. If the shoulders are tight, it's likely that the strap muscles in the neck that connect to the shoulders are also tight.

At least the child can touch these muscles and even see what it looks like when you contract some of these muscles. For example, the strap muscles in the neck may bulge as you tense them. You can freeze your shoulders and show the child how they won't freely move when they are tight. You can demonstrate what it looks like and sounds like to talk through a clenched jaw or with tight lips. Talk with the child about how tension in any of these areas can alter how the voice and speech sounds.

See if the child can identify where he is exhibiting excess tension. You might have him look in the mirror to see if his shoulders are elevated or if his jaw appears tight. You can even gently massage the muscles of the shoulders or back of the neck to see if that feels tight to the child.

Identifying excess muscle tension in the respiratory muscles

If the child has excess tension in the respiratory muscles, he will probably be breathing in a shallow way, using the muscles of the upper chest instead of the diaphragm. Refer to Chapter 7 (pages 101-115) for more information on explaining respiration to the child.

Reducing muscle tension

	Child will use techniques to reduce muscle tension in:
HF Treatment Objective 3	a. phonatory muscles b. oro-pharyngeal musculature c. respiratory muscles

Now that the child is able to tell where he is exhibiting too much tension, he has to learn techniques to reduce the tension in non-speech tasks. This will allow the child to move to the next step: learning how to maintain this more relaxed state while phonating in speech tasks of increasing length (See Treatment Objective #4, page 73). Although this book describes the techniques for reducing tension related to the three areas (phonatory, oro-pharyngeal, and respiratory), you must integrate the techniques for a holistic approach. You'll need the child to concentrate on breathing while practicing relaxed phonation. If there is tension in the oro-pharyngeal region, the child will need to coordinate breathing, phonation, and relaxed muscles in the face and neck, for example. In fact, you may want to approach these in reverse order from what is listed here. That is, first start with assuring the child is breathing appropriately, then address tension in the oro-pharyngeal area (described by Verdolini in Hillman & Verdolini, 1999) as *deactivation,* and then move to what she calls *activation,* or phonation as described here.

Reducing muscle tension of the phonatory muscles

Because different children will respond better to one technique or another, a variety of techniques are described. Don't jump from one to another. Be sure to give one technique an adequate trial before selecting another. These exercises may seem odd to the child. You'll need to provide adequate verbal descriptions, but most importantly you must be able to model the technique. You must find a technique that works easily for the child because you'll use this technique to advance the child to using easy phonation into words, phrases, sentences, and conversation. These techniques are described in Appendix 5B (page 80) and can be sent home with the child for practice.

1. Yawn-sigh (Boone 1971)

The *yawn-sigh* is one of the facilitating techniques first described by Boone in 1971. Explain to the child that when he yawns, his mouth opens wide, his tongue drops to the floor of his mouth, and his soft palate lifts. Tell the child to imagine that a balloon is being blown up inside his mouth. These changes occur not only in the oral cavity, but there is an expansion of the upper airway as well. This means that the muscles of the mouth and the throat are opening and relaxing. Have the child practice yawning several times. Then ask the child to make a very quiet, unforced sound on the exhalation after the yawn. This is the sigh. Demonstrate the easy, relaxed sigh you are seeking. To make this more challenging, you can ask the child to vary the sigh. That is, ask the child to make the pitch of the sigh sound go up and down. This sigh can later be shaped into words beginning with "h" or with a vowel sound.

2. Inhalation phonation

This is also one of Boone's facilitating techniques. It is useful because the sound made on inhalation can only be made by the true vocal folds. Therefore, if you know that the child is exhibiting lateral compression with squeezing of the ventricular folds, this technique can help the child get the feel of phonation made with the true vocal folds.

Explain to the child that people usually make sound when they are exhaling but you're going to try a technique that's backwards. That is, you're going to have the child make a sound as he breathes in. You may want to place your hand on your abdomen as you demonstrate this so the child associates the movement of your hand, indicating you are breathing in, with the production of the sound. (See Chapter 7, pages 101-107, for more information on respiration.) Have the child imitate this with you several times. Since the child is used to inhaling through his nose, the sound will be similar to a hum, and will sound high-pitched.

The next step is to have the child inhale and make the high-pitched humming sound, and then continue the sound on the exhalation. If the quality of the phonation changes significantly on the exhalation, the child has probably gone back to a hyperfunctional production. Practice making the sound on inhalation and continuing the sound on exhalation until the quality sounds the same. It is ideal if there is not a break in phonation at the peak of inhalation, when exhalation begins.

When the child has mastered this, ask him to change the sound he is making on exhalation so that it sweeps down from the high-pitched sound into the more normal register. It will continue to be a humming sound.

Then ask the child to inhale without making a sound and try making the high-pitched humming sound on exhalation. If at any time the child reverts to the tense phonation, return to using phonation on the inhalation and exhalation. When the child can make a sound on exhalation only, and can drop it into the more normal register, this technique can be used to shape production of words, phrases, etc. You can help prepare the child for this by asking him to open his mouth and "let a vowel sound come out" at the end of the exhalation. You can then have the child begin to vary the parameters of that vowel sound. That is, the child can make the pitch go up and down, or change the loudness.

3. Achieving relaxed phonation through front focus sounds
A review of several methods finds similar descriptions stressing the importance of teaching the child to produce an easy phonation that is focused in the nasal cavity and toward the front of the face. The *Accent Method* (Kotby et al. 1991, Kotby 1995), Stemple's *Vocal Function Exercises* (1994), and Verdolini's *Resonant Voice Therapy* (1998) as well as Rammage's (1996) self-help guide for patients all describe techniques to get the child producing a humming, buzzing sound in the nose or on the lips. This focus in the nasopharynx helps the child shift focus from the tension that has been placed in the laryngeal area. Some of these techniques are described in Chapter 9, pages 137-146, related to improving tone focus.

Have the child produce "hmmmm" in a very relaxed way. Listen carefully to see if the child is producing this with a clear voice and no tension. This is described in Verdolini as the basic training gesture. Stemple, instead, uses a nasalized production of the vowel sound "ee." This may be a bit harder for the child than producing the "hmm" in the nasal cavity.

Then have the child take this same sound and begin to vary the pitch. Rammage calls this the *vocal siren*. If you use this term with the child, make sure he understands that you don't mean loud like a siren but made in the front of the mouth so it sounds like a siren. At first, pitch variations will be very small, but as the child gains confidence with this type of phonation, the pitch variations will increase.

Instead of pitch variations that go up and down and up and down, Stemple has the child go from the lowest note to the highest note. Both he and Rammage suggest that a raspberry (made with the lips) is a good sound for this because it keeps the focus of the sound at the front of the face. Rammage has the child use this vocal siren with other continuant sounds like "rrrrr" and "hnnnn" or even "hng."

After the child has mastered maintaining easy phonation on one of these vocal gestures (e.g., "hmm," "ee," raspberry), resonant voice therapy uses something called a *chant hierarchy*. The child is asked to make variations between the voiced "m" and a voiceless sound "p" to be sure that the child can ease back into phonation on the next voiced consonant. Therefore, the child is asked to repeat the sequence "me-pee-me-pee-me-pee-me-pee" maintaining relaxed phonation.

The next step in the hierarchy is to have the child practice the vocal gesture with pitch and loudness variations. That is, have the child repeat "me-pee-me-pee-me-pee-me-pee," getting louder and softer, going up and down in pitch, and even combining those two aspects.

After the child has mastered these different steps for producing the relaxed tone focused in the nose in front of the mouth, you will be able to shape this into production of words and phrases.

Reducing muscle tension in the oro-pharyngeal muscles

Reducing muscle tension in the muscles of the face, mouth, neck, and shoulders can be a very fun part of therapy. The exercises and stretches to accomplish this are also fairly easy for parents to practice at home. As mentioned above, reducing tension in the area should occur before beginning phonatory exercises. You may want to start each therapy session with a review of some of these exercises, based on where you have identified tension for this particular child. Does the child carry tension in the jaw, lips, tongue, neck and/or shoulders? Select the stretches and exercises to target those areas.

These stretches are described in Appendix 5C, pages 81-82, which can be used as a homework sheet. They have been drawn from Boone (1971), Stemple (1994), Verdolini (1998), and Rammage (1996). Any exercises involving the neck should be done gently. Never force a movement and never perform the movement if it is painful.

Reducing muscle tension when breathing

If there is excess muscle tension when breathing, the child is probably breathing using the upper chest and shoulders. Chapter 7, pages 104-105, explains exercises that will help the child establish a pattern of diaphragmatic breathing.

Transferring the new relaxed phonation into speech

HF Treatment Objective 4	Child will use techniques to eliminate muscle tension during: a. words and phrases b. sentences c. conversation

A combination of the approaches to reduced muscle tension in the phonatory, oro-pharyngeal, and respiratory muscles should result in the child producing relaxed-sounding phonation on some vocal gestures (e.g., "hmm," "eee") and varying pitch and loudness. Don't rush the child, but when he seems to have good mastery at that level, begin to introduce words and phrases. If the child is using a nasal sound ("m" or "n"), you may want to try words that begin with those sounds (see Appendix 9B, pages 148-149, and choose words from the sentences for practice). You can also try words that begin with vowel sounds (see Appendix 8F, page 131). If you use the *yawn-sigh*, the child might have the most success with words beginning with "h" (see Appendix 8I, page 134). Gradually help the child produce longer and longer utterances with the new, easy phonatory pattern.

Summary

Since most voice disorders have some component of hyperfunction, understanding the physiology causing a hyperfunctional voice disorder is important. An instrumental evaluation of the voice including visualization will help define the type of hyperfunction. Careful treatment planning with a combination of techniques will help the child achieve a healthy voice.

Relaxed Phonation vs. Strained Phonation

Use these pictures to discriminate between tense and appropriate function.

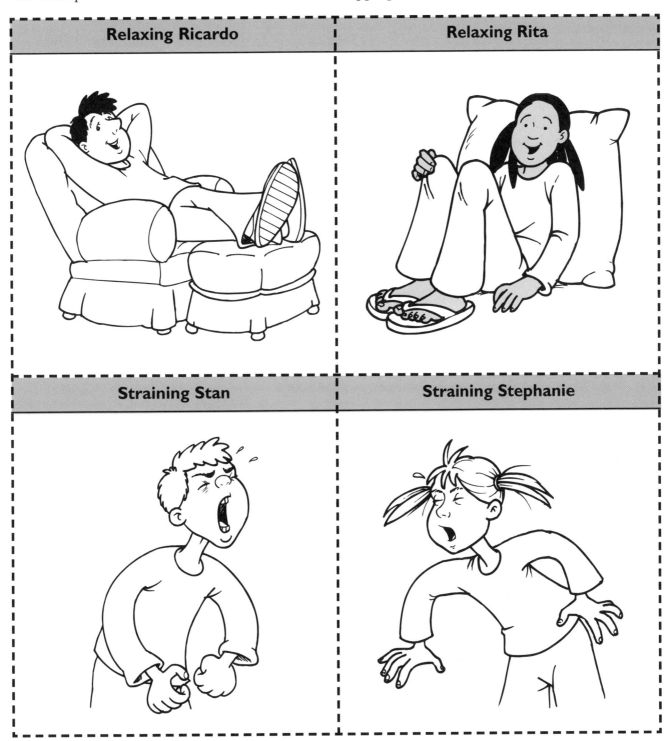

Relaxing Ricardo

Relaxing Rita

Straining Stan

Straining Stephanie

79

Reducing Tension in the Phonatory Muscles

❑ **Yawn-sigh**
Open your mouth wide as you yawn. Make a soft "sigh" when the air comes out after the yawn. Make sure you're not forcing the sound and that it sounds very relaxed.

❑ **Inhalation Phonation**
Keeping your lips lightly closed, breathe in through your nose, making a sound as you breathe in. This humming sound will probably be high-pitched. Then make the same sound as you breathe out.

❑ **Front focus sounds**
Take a nice breath in and make the sound "hmmm" as you breathe out. Be sure the sound is not forced and that it is very relaxed.

Follow the steps that have been marked.

_____ Make your sound go up and down in pitch just a little bit.

_____ Make your sound go up and down more in pitch.

_____ Make your sound get louder and then softer, then louder.

mmme-pee-me-pee

_____ If you need to, use your sound to get started. Then repeat "me-pee-me-pee-me-pee."

_____ Repeat "me-pee-me-pee-me-pee" and make your pitch go up and down.

mmme   me   me
    pee   pee

_____ Repeat "me-pee-me-pee-me-pee" and make it louder-softer-louder-softer.

ME-pee-ME-pee

Reducing Tension in the Oro-Pharyngeal Muscles

Repeat each marked exercise _____ times. Complete this practice _____ times a day.

Shoulders

Shoulder shrugs
Pull the shoulders up around your ears and feel the tension. Hold for a few seconds. Then let all the tension go as your shoulders drop down.

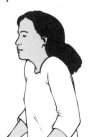

Shoulder rolls
Make big circles with your shoulders. Have them go up by your ears, then back, down, then forward and up to your ears again. Reverse direction.

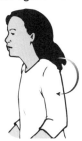

Neck

Head pull side to side
Reach your right hand over your head to the left side. Pull your head gently toward the right and hold for a few seconds. Reverse and do with the other hand.

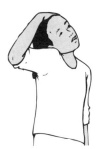

Head turns
Keep your head straight and look to the right as you try to see over your shoulder. Hold for a few seconds. Reverse direction.

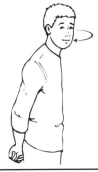

Head sweep
Drop your chin to your chest. Keep your chin on your chest and slowly turn your head to the right. Look up and over your shoulder. Hold for a few seconds.. Slowly sweep your chin back down to the middle of your chest. Reverse direction.

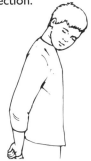

Head drop
Stand up. Let your head drop forward with your chin on your chest. Hold this position for 10-20 seconds to stretch the muscles in the back of your neck.

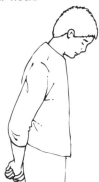

Jaw

Jaw stretch (with y of hand)
Make a "y" with your hand. Gently pull your jaw open and hold it.

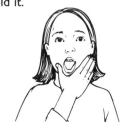

Jaw molding (with heel)
Use the heel of your hand to gently massage your jaw open.

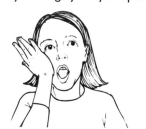

Chewing gum
Pretend to chew gum. Exaggerate the movements of your jaw.

Lips

Raspberries
Blow a raspberry with your lips.

Loose lips
Pretend your lips are numb and you can't squeeze them together tightly. Make the "puh-puh-puh-puh" sound with lots of air coming out.

Tongue

Tongue out
Open your jaw wide and stick your tongue way out. Say "haaa."

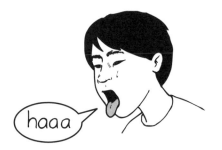

haaa

Back and forth (huh-yuh-huh-yuh)
Hold your jaw steady. Move your tongue all the way back and then out as far as it can go. Add a sound. Say "huh" when your tongue is out and "yuh" when your tongue is back.

Tongue trill
This is like a raspberry but made with the tongue. It's a very fast "t" sound made by blowing the air past the tongue.

Ta-ta-ta-ta
Stick your tongue out of your mouth and make the sound "ta-ta-ta."

Combined

Goalpost yawn
Put your arms out like a goalpost and move them back and forth a little. At the same time, open wide, yawn, and turn your head from side to side.

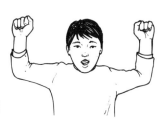

Rag doll
Stand up. Lean over with your head and arms hanging down. Slowly come up by first straightening your lower back, then your middle back, and then your shoulders. The last thing to come up is your head.

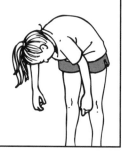

6   Treatment for Vocal Abuse

The most common reason children have voice problems is vocal abuse, also called *poor vocal hygiene*. In fact, *vocal abuse* (poor vocal hygiene) and *good vocal hygiene* are opposites. As you work with the child to eliminate behaviors that are abusive to the voice, you will help the child substitute good vocal hygiene behaviors, helping to maintain a healthy vocal mechanism. You can also teach the child vocal hygiene behaviors that are good for anyone's voice, whether or not they are replacing an unacceptable behavior. (The PowerPoint presentation, pages 169-172 and on the CD, has more information on vocal abuse and vocal hygiene.)

Convincing a child to reduce or eliminate vocally abusive behaviors is difficult, and for some children it is impossible. Use the information provided in Chapter 5 (pages 70-82) as you meet with the child and the child's parents to discuss the results of the evaluation and to make sure everyone is in agreement that therapy should proceed. Use the lesson plans and activities in this chapter to try to change as many of the abusive behaviors as possible. If the child is compliant with vocal abuse reduction, a change in vocal quality should be observed within a few months. If there is a laryngeal pathology (e.g., nodules), there should also be a significant change or elimination of the nodules in that amount of time.

Short-term Goal

Child will eliminate abusive vocal behaviors. (VA)

Treatment Objectives

1. Child will identify vocally abusive behaviors. (VA-1)

2. Child will collect reliable baseline data on abusive behaviors. (VA-2)

3. Child will identify acceptable alternatives to vocally abusive behaviors. (VA-3)

4. Child will reduce/eliminate the following abusive behaviors: _____. (VA-4)

5. Child will substitute acceptable alternatives for vocally abusive behaviors. (VA-5)

Note: If the child is also misusing the voice, add appropriate activities from Chapters 7-9 (pages 101-156). It is possible that the child may also demonstrate hyperfunction of the vocal mechanism and will require techniques described in Chapter 5.

Specific Lessons to Teach

Use the information provided in the following lessons in any way that works best for the child. Depending on the length and frequency of the sessions, age and motivation of the child, and setting in which the services are provided, you may choose to teach only one lesson each time you see the child. However, it is more likely that you will combine information from several lessons into one treatment session. For example, your first session might include helping the child identify vocal abuses and selecting some good vocal hygiene techniques. The homework might involve activities to increase the child's awareness of the frequency of one or more of the abuses.

Identifying vocal abuses

VA Treatment Objective 1	Child will identify vocally abusive behaviors.

By this time, you have already spoken with the child in general terms to explain the voice disorder and your general plan of treatment. You and the child and parent have already agreed on the behavior reinforcement system and whether the child will be earning tokens for a "big prize." (Note: In almost all instances, it will be necessary to have the child working for a big prize.) The first lesson focuses on helping the child very specifically describe what she is doing with her voice that is hurting her voice.

Getting specific about vocal abuses

Use Appendix 6A, page 93, to help the child identify the ways that she is hurting her voice. Discuss each of the possible abuses and help the child decide if she does or does not use her voice in that way. If the child indicates that she uses a vocal abuse, discuss the *why* and the *when*. A discussion of why the child uses her voice in this way is likely to involve talking about emotions and how we handle emotions. Remember that at different ages, children have different levels of awareness of emotions and how to express them (see Chapter 5, pages 70-82). Failing to address psychodynamic issues (e.g., aggressive behavior) that prompt voice abuse is likely to sabotage your efforts to change the child's voice use.

While helping the child complete the *When* column, elicit all the different instances during which the child might use this vocal behavior. For example, if the child indicates she talks loudly over noise and provides one example of talking over the television, try to elicit other examples. Does she talk to her parent in the kitchen while the dishwasher is running? Does she talk to her brother while the dog is barking? The more specific you can get the child to be, the easier it will be to target situations in which the behavior can be reduced or eliminated.

Getting help from others

Some children are better historians than others. Some children can tell you very specifically the kinds of things they do with their voices and when and where they occur. Other children may seem totally unaware of any vocally abusive behaviors and may not be able to give you much information about when the abuses occur. You may need to rely on the child's parents, teachers, coaches, and others to gather the specific information you need about vocally abusive behaviors.

Identifying potential targets for change

After identifying as many vocal abuses as possible, determine the frequency of each abuse and the potential for change. Those behaviors that occur the most frequently will have the biggest impact on the voice if eliminated. However, you must also consider which behaviors are most likely to change. For example, if the child has a medical problem causing coughing, trying to eliminate the coughing may not be reasonable. Also be sure to include any problematic interpersonal behaviors that need to be addressed such as excessively loud talking used to gain attention or excessive crying when interacting with siblings.

Increasing awareness of frequency of vocal abuse

VA Treatment Objective 2	Child will collect reliable baseline data on abusive behaviors.

Even the astute child who has been able to accurately identify abuses of the voice may not be aware of the number of times that a particular abuse occurs throughout the day. After you identify a single form of abuse or several forms of abuse that you want the child to reduce or eliminate, it may be necessary to heighten the child's awareness of when the abuses are occurring. Decide whether you will address one or more than one abuse based on the child's understanding of the problem, age, motivation, and any other factors that will impact the child's chance of success.

Obtaining baseline data

Increasing the child's awareness and obtaining baseline data can be accomplished at the same time. This requires the cooperation and participation of adults with whom the child interacts. For young children, the adult may have to assume the responsibility for both pointing out the abuse and recording the data for baseline information. In some cases, the adult may have to point out the occurrence of the abuse, but the child might then assume the responsibility for recording that data. An older child may be able to perform both functions. That is, once the particular type of abuse is pointed out to the child, she may do a very good job identifying when it happens and then be able to record the data.

Accuracy in identifying abusive behaviors

Some abusive behaviors are fairly easy for the child and other adults to identify. For example, everyone probably agrees on what a scream is. However if something more subjective, such as talking too loudly, has been identified as an abuse, it is likely you'll need to train both the child and the adults who will be helping to monitor the behavior on exactly what loud talking is. Some of the interpersonal behaviors may be difficult for the child to notice. If she has always had poor listening skills, for example, she is not likely to notice now when she is exhibiting this behavior. The child must also understand that you want accurate data. Any small reinforcement given (see Chapter 4, pages 42-69) is contingent upon accurate and honest data collection.

Selecting time periods for data collection

It's an impossible task for the child to pay attention to abuses and collect baseline data throughout an entire day. Therefore it is helpful if you define specific times during which you would like the baseline data collected. Based on the information the child has provided to you about when the abuses occur, select a period of time during which you could expect a high frequency of occurrence. It is helpful if you select several different types of situations in which to collect baseline data, including some that address the interpersonal skills you have identified. For example, if the child indicates she screams at her brother at bedtime, at her teammates at soccer practice, and on the playground, you may want to have the child collect baseline data in each of these situations. This will require that you gain the cooperation and assistance from the parents, the coach, and the teacher. At the end of the prescribed period of time, the adult records the total number of occurrences of abuse on the data collection form. You can collect only one type of abuse (e.g., throat clearing, see chart at right) over multiple days or use the form to collect data on all abuses that occur during those time periods. When collecting data on multiple abuses (e.g., screaming, throat clearing, coughing to get attention, loud singing), you may want to use a different chart each day or use different colored ink on the same chart.

If you have identified several specific situations as problematic, you can chart the occurrence of the behaviors only in those situations over a period of days. For example, you could have the child's coach record screaming at soccer practice on the two nights of practice and game day on one chart and the parents record making loud noises at home on another.

Chart to Collect Baseline Data on Vocal Abuse			
Name Theo Throat Clearer			
Date/Time period	Location or activity	Undesirable behaviors 👎	Recorder
Thursday 6:30-7	Breakfast	⊞	Mom
Friday 9-11	Classroom	IIII	Social Studies Teacher
Saturday 12-2	Basketball game	⊞ I	Older sister
Sunday 10-11	Sunday School Class	⊞ III	Teacher
Monday 11-11:45	Lunch room	⊞ I	Classroom aide
Tuesday 3-5	Homework clinic	⊞	Teacher

(See Appendix 6B, page 94, for a blank form.)

Using a signal

Most children will respond negatively if their peers know that the child is being monitored for doing something "wrong" with her voice. Therefore, if the adult is responsible for pointing out the occurrences of abuse, it's a good idea if the adult and the child agree upon a signal that will be known only to them. For example, the adult could quietly touch her throat, snap her fingers, or even say a code word (e.g., "there" or "got it").

Easy ways to tally

If the child is assuming responsibility for identifying when the abuses occur, it may be helpful if the child has an easy way to keep the tally during the designated period of time. In certain situations, this may be as easy as providing the child with a small pad of paper. For example, if the child is collecting information about the number of times she talks too loudly in class, she can record it on the pad. However, if the child is monitoring a behavior that occurs in a less structured situation, such as yelling on the playground, it is not viable to expect the child to carry around a pad of paper. Sporting goods stores typically have stroke counters used by golfers that the child may enjoy using. Some are worn on the wrist and others fit in a pocket. Many models are under $5, but there are more elaborate electronic models for around $20.

Keeping up with tally sheets and involving the child

Regardless of the age of the child, as much responsibility as possible should be placed on the child. This keeps the child vested in the process and increases awareness of the number of times the abuse is occurring. Even in a young child who cannot be responsible for writing on the tally sheet, she can at least be responsible for keeping track of the tally sheets themselves. The child might collect the tally sheet from the adult at the end of the period of time and remember to give it to the next adult for the subsequent prescribed data collection period.

Recording cumulative baseline data

When the baseline data is reported to you (typically for a period of a week), transfer it to a graph or chart to help the child better see the total number of abuses tallied at baseline. Depending on the frequency of the abuse, you can use a graph in several ways. You can tally the total number of abuses or the single targeted abuse for the entire week from the data sheets the child turns in. (See Appendix 6C, page 95, for a blank graph.)

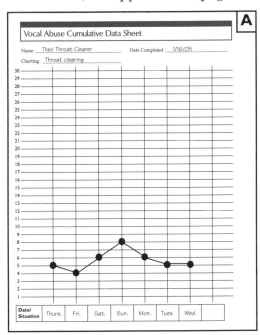 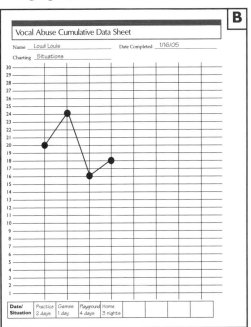

If it is a single targeted abuse, as in example A, you probably won't have to go very far up the vertical axis. If the child had been collecting data on all abuses throughout the day, you might need the higher numbers. You could also chart abuses according to the situations rather than by days (example B). The child might bring in one chart for practice/games, a second chart for playground, and a third chart for home.

Whatever you decide, you must be consistent when you collect subsequent data for comparison to determine if frequency is decreasing. That is, if baseline data was collected for four hours total a day and in specific situations, you will want to sample those same situations for the same length of time in subsequent data collection. If the child is monitoring several different kinds of vocal abuse in several different situations, she might have a variety of graphs on which you are documenting frequency. You might have a graph for throat clearing by day for a week and another for crying by day for the week. Use your judgment to determine how much data the child can collect reliably and how much graphing and charting the child can understand. These same graphs will be used throughout therapy to record future tally sheets that hopefully will reflect a decrease in the frequency of the behavior.

Identifying alternatives to vocal abuses

VA Treatment Objective 3	Child will identify acceptable alternatives to vocally abusive behaviors

Asking the child to eliminate a behavior without substituting a different behavior will likely lead to failure. Appendix 6D, pages 96-97, will be helpful in your discussions with the child as you contrast behaviors that are harmful to the voice and those that are not. Since yelling and screaming are probably the most frequent vocal abuses demonstrated by children, the appendix lists several different alternatives for yelling and screaming. You may need to explain how some of these behaviors make a sound but don't really use the voice. For example, it may seem confusing to the child that a loud "ssss" sound can be made without harming the voice. You and the child may come up with many other creative alternatives to voice abuse. Not only do these ideas need to be interesting, they need to be doable in a variety of situations. For example, stomping your feet may be acceptable in the bleachers at a sporting event but certainly not for gaining the teacher's attention in the classroom. The adults who interact with the child need to be made aware of any alternative behaviors so that the adults respond appropriately.

Include a discussion of any interpersonal skills that are leading to vocal abuse and alternatives to these behaviors and feelings. Appendix 6E, page 98, may help guide your discussion. You may wish to seek the assistance of a school guidance counselor or psychologist if the child has significant interpersonal and psychodynamic factors to be addressed.

Since coughing and throat clearing are two very common abuses, some discussion of alternative behaviors is warranted. As noted in Chapter 1, a child may cough or clear the throat because she has a sensation that there is something in her throat. The easiest alternative behavior to use is a forceful swallow. Stemple et al. (2000) calls this a *hard swallow*. Explain to the child that she probably feels like something is in her throat and that feeling makes her want to clear her throat (or cough). If the cough/throat clear is related to a vocal pathology, like nodules, explain to the child that no amount of throat clearing will make the nodules and the sensation disappear. In fact, the throat clearing will only make it worse. Suggest that a hard swallow will help to relieve the sensation and if there is anything (e.g., mucous) on the vocal folds, the swallow will help clear it. You can use the picture from Appendix 4A, page 54, to show the child how swallowing might send whatever is on the vocal folds down to the stomach.

If the child insists that something is on the vocal folds (and there may be mucous there), teach the child to use a silent cough (Zwitman et al. 1973). You can explain it by telling the child to make a big "h" sound followed by a swallow. Explain that the "h" uses only air, no vibration of the vocal folds. Show the child the picture of the lungs and their relationship to the voice box and to the esophagus. You might even blow up a balloon and show how a forceful squeeze to the balloon shoots the air up past the opening. That is what a big "h" sound does—blows air forcefully past the vocal folds, blowing off anything sitting on the folds that is then swallowed. The child should be instructed to take a big breath, forcefully produce the "h" sound, and then swallow. This silent cough should be used only when a swallow won't relieve the sensation and only if you are convinced that it really is productive (i.e., clearing mucous from the folds).

After you and the child have identified the problem behaviors and interaction skills and selected appropriate alternatives, complete Appendix 6F, page 99. For the younger child, you could draw in pictures (or cut and paste pictures from Appendix 6D in the columns. Older children can just write to fill in the columns.

Reducing abuses/substituting alternative behaviors

VA Treatment Objective 4	Child will reduce/eliminate the following abusive behaviors: _____.

VA Treatment Objective 5	Child will substitute acceptable alternatives for vocally abusive behaviors.

After you and the child have identified the vocally abusive behaviors to change and collected baseline data on each, you are ready to establish a program to help the child eliminate, or at least significantly reduce, the frequency of these abusive behaviors. You also want the child to substitute other more acceptable vocal behaviors.

Select one or more of the behaviors and determine the period of time or activity during which you want the child to monitor and reduce the behavior. If the child is learning to substitute a more acceptable behavior for an abusive behavior, the child might tally both. If there are no alternative behaviors, you can cross out that column. Provide the data collection sheet (See Appendix 6G, page 100, for a blank chart) and a counter if the child is responsible for counting occurrences. Instruct the child how and when to fill out the sheet.

Chart to Record Behaviors to Reduce and Substitute

Name: Fifi Funnysounds

Date/Time period	Target behaviors 👍 Quiet voice Coming into room to talk Not talking on low air	Undesirable behaviors 👎 Throat clearing Yelling Making animal noises Using voice to get attention	Recorder
April 10th Noon–2:00	✓ ✓ ✓ ✓ ✓ ✓ ✓ ✓	x x x x	Preschool teacher
April 10th 6:00–6:30	✓ ✓ ✓ Remembered to come to the kitchen to talk to Mom	x x Yelled at brother who was stealing her dessert	Mom
April 10th 8:00–9:00	✓ ✓ Used quiet voice when working on homework	x Throat clearing after toothbrushing	Dad
April 11th 7:30–8:00	✓ ✓ Talked quietly with brother in car on way to school	x x Yelled at brother when getting out of car; yelled to get attention of friend on school steps	Dad
April 11th 10:00–10:30	✓ ✓ ✓ Walked up to teacher's desk to ask question; talked quietly to students at table	x x Demonstrated sound animal makes that she was drawing; yelled "Hey teacher" from back of room to get attention	Art teacher

If at all possible, have the child take responsibility for counting the behaviors, as self-monitoring has been shown to be effective in learning to control the behavior (Miller 1980, Johnson 1985). Johnson points out that self-monitoring brings the behaviors to a conscious level. The fact that the child then has to record the behavior means she has encountered a consequence for that behavior. Though not terribly time-consuming, having to record the behavior is almost a punishment. Punishment is known to decrease the occurrence of a behavior.

Be sure the child knows that you will reinforce her for turning in accurate data. If you place too much emphasis on rewarding a decrease in the behaviors, the child may artificially decrease the numbers. Having an adult help monitor the child's tally may increase accuracy.

The child should bring the tally sheet to each therapy session. Record the data on Appendix 6C (page 95) and provide a reinforcement for accurate data collection. Discuss with the child what a reasonable goal might be for the next period of time (i.e., between therapy sessions). If you have only been targeting one behavior, you might add a second one so that the child is responsible for monitoring and changing more than one behavior during the next period.

If the child is having a hard time getting all the data recorded or isn't receiving close enough supervision to help maintain motivation, suggest that the child report data daily by phone. Set a prescribed time each day for the child to call in a report. This does not mean you have to take a daily call from the child. You can have the child leave the information on an answering machine or with voice mail. The child might also fill out a pre-stamped postcard at the end of each day and drop it in the mail to you. Computer-savvy children may enjoy sending you a daily e-mail message with their data.

Practicing alternative behaviors

So what else goes on during the therapy session besides charting the data the child reports? The child should be engaged in activities to practice the alternative behaviors. Role-playing situations (e.g., you pretend to be the child's sibling or teammate) will allow the child to gain confidence with the use of the new skills. Role play is especially useful when addressing psychodynamic factors, including interpersonal skills.

Transferring skills

To help the child transfer the skills, you might accompany her to problematic situations. You could sit in on one of the classes where she tends to exhibit the abusive behavior, such as gym class. You might meet her at swim practice or go to the playground for recess. You can also invite other children into the therapy session. If the child has particular difficulty interacting with a friend or sibling, arrange to have that child attend a therapy session. You can also ask one of the child's friends to help the child monitor behavior outside the therapy room. Invite the friend to therapy and enlist her help. She can be the child's "secret voice buddy" in problem situations.

Vocal Hygiene

As you continue to help the child reduce or eliminate problem vocal behaviors, you may also need to teach the child about other good vocal hygiene habits that are helpful for anyone's voice. These habits do not need to be replacing any particular abuse. *Hygiene* is probably not a familiar word to many children, so you may want to call these "healthy voice habits." The child should understand that these behaviors are good for everyone's voice and once adopted, should be things she does forever. Some of these healthy voice habits may already have been identified as alternative behaviors. You can find more information about vocal hygiene in the PowerPoint presentation on pages 169-172 and on the accompanying CD.

Short-term Goal

Child will adopt good vocal hygiene techniques. (VH)

Treatment Objectives

1. Child will drink water to keep vocal mechanism hydrated. (VH-1)

2. Child will get an adequate amount of sleep. (VH-2)

3. Child will avoid beverages and food with caffeine. (VH-3)

4. Child will avoid exposure to smoke/chemicals. (VH-4)

5. Child will use an acceptable volume. (VH-5)

6. Child will speak to others from an appropriate distance. (VH-6)

VH Treatment Objective 1	Child will drink water to keep vocal mechanism hydrated.

It is generally accepted that keeping the vocal mechanism moist helps to maintain a healthy voice. It is thought that hydration treatments (e.g., drinking water, using humidifiers, taking mucolytic drugs) help reduce edema-based lesions (Verdolini-Marston 1991, Verdolini-Marston et al. 1994). Verdolini-Marston et al. (1994) and Stemple et al. (2000) point out that in order to use a mechanism that is not well hydrated, the child probably has to use more pressure to phonate. This behavior may lead to fatigue of the voice or even vocal pathologies. The best way to maintain hydration is for the child to drink a lot of water. You may need to explain that the water doesn't directly touch the vocal folds, but when the whole body is better hydrated, the secretory glands in the laryngeal ventricles can lubricate the vocal folds (Stemple et al. 2000).

You might use an analogy with props to help the child understand why hydration is important. Show the child a new rubber band and demonstrate how easily it vibrates when pulled. Then show the child an old, cracked rubber band and explain that this is what the vocal folds might look like if we don't drink enough water. Demonstrate how this rubber band doesn't vibrate well.

Getting enough sleep

VH Treatment Objective 2	Child will get an adequate amount of sleep.

Since most children's bedtimes are controlled by the parents, this may be a message you need to communicate with them. If a child is tired all the time, she may use a lower pitch or a more gravelly vocal quality and fail to project her voice. She may also be too tired to remember other good vocal behaviors being taught.

Avoiding caffeine

VH Treatment Objective 3	Child will avoid beverages and food with caffeine.

Though few children drink coffee, they may still be ingesting quite a bit of caffeine by drinking soft drinks with caffeine and by eating chocolate. Caffeine dries the mucous membranes. This message can be tied to the information about increasing hydration with water. When trying to eliminate caffeine, the child may be more successful with a gradual withdrawal.

Avoiding exposure to smoke and other chemicals

VH Treatment Objective 4	Child will avoid exposure to smoke/chemicals.

If the child lives in a household where an adult smokes, you should meet with the parent to discuss the deleterious effects of secondhand smoke related to voice production. A child with a voice problem should not be around smoke or other chemical airborne irritants.

Using an acceptable volume

VH Treatment Objective 5	Child will use an acceptable volume.

Children can be taught to monitor the volume they use to talk in different situations (see Chapter 8, pages 117-120). If the child is typically a "loud talker," enlist the help of adults in the child's environment to increase the child's awareness of how loudly she is talking.

Avoiding talking from room to room

VH Treatment Objective 6	Child will speak to others from an appopriate distance.

A good rule of thumb is to teach the child that she should be close enough to touch the person to whom she is speaking. This will help the child understand that it is not a good idea to stand at the top of the stairs to talk to a sibling at the bottom or to carry on a conversation from the family room when her dad is in the kitchen.

Summary

If the child's voice problem is solely related to poor vocal hygiene (vocal abuse), then the activities in this chapter should provide the information needed to remediate the problem. If the child is misusing other aspects (e.g., respiration, onset, pitch), then you'll need to integrate information from later chapters.

If you want more detailed information about how to implement a vocal abuse reduction program, you might consult resources like those listed on page 173 that provide more step-by-step instructions and forms.

Things I Do That Hurt My Voice

Put a star by those behaviors you want to change.

Things that hurt voices	I do this	I don't do this	Why I do this	When and how often I do this
yelling/screaming				
loud laughing				
loud crying				
too much crying				
coughing				
clearing my throat				
cheering				
talking loudly				
talking over noise				
making funny noises				
loud whispering				
using my voice all the time				
trying to get attention ⋆				
Others:				
Others:				

Appendix 6A
The Source for Children's Voice Disorders

Chart to Collect Baseline Data on Vocal Abuse

Name _____

Date/Time period	Location or activity	Undesirable behaviors	Recorder

Vocal Abuse Cumulative Data Sheet

Name _____ Date Completed _____

Charting _____

30									
29									
28									
27									
26									
25									
24									
23									
22									
21									
20									
19									
18									
17									
16									
15									
14									
13									
12									
11									
10									
9									
8									
7									
6									
5									
4									
3									
2									
1									
Date/ Situation									

Appendix 6C
The Source for Children's Voice Disorders

Things I Can Try Instead of Using My Voice

Instead of		I can try this	
Screaming/yelling when I am mad		• clapping • making a loud "ssss" • stomping my feet • throwing a tissue at the wall • puffing up my cheeks and blowing air • jumping quietly up and down • telling the person very quietly why I am mad	
Yelling to gain someone's attention		• clapping • snapping fingers • ringing a bell • whistling • using baby monitors or walkie-talkies	
Loud laughing		• quiet laughing	
Loud crying		• quiet crying • sad or pouty face	
Too much crying		• less crying • sad or pouty face	
Coughing		• swallowing • silent cough	

Instead of	I can try this
Clearing my throat	• swallowing • silent cough
Cheering	• clapping • stomping my feet • using noisemakers
Talking loudly	• using my inside voice • going close to the person to talk • using baby monitors or walkie-talkies
Talking over noise	• turning off the noise • moving somewhere else to talk
Making funny noises	• keeping a quiet voice • making a funny face
Loud whispering	• going close to the person to talk
Talking all the time	• talking less

Things I Can Do to Interact Better with Others

Instead of	I can try this
Talking too much	Counting to 10 in my head before talking
Not taking turns	Remembering I don't have to go first
Not paying attention to others	Listening and retelling what I've been told when they tell me something
Trying to get people to pay attention to me	Pretending to be a fly hiding on the wall
Not listening	Touching my listening stone in my pocket
Not changing my behavior to match the situation	Paying attention to how others are acting and talking

Appendix 6E
The Source for Children's Voice Disorders

Things I Can Do Instead That Won't Hurt My Voice

Now I do this and it hurts my voice.	I can do this instead.

Chart to Record Behaviors to Reduce and Substitute

Name _____

Date/Time period	Target behaviors 👍	Undesirable behaviors 👎	Recorder

Appendix 6G
The Source for Children's Voice Disorders

7 Treatment for Respiration

Why work on respiration?

Many children already use adequate respiratory support for both their speaking and their singing voices. Your clinical evaluation will have revealed any abnormal breathing patterns (e.g., excessive movement of the upper chest indicating clavicular breathing). If it appears that the child is not using adequate respiratory support or a good pattern of breathing, then it is important to address respiration. Stemple et al. (2000, p. 291) state that "respiratory training, whether direct or indirect, is a primary part of improving the disordered voice." As Stemple et al. further explain, most therapy techniques address air pressures and airflow to help the child produce a more efficient voice. This requires achieving a good balance between respiration, phonation, and resonance. The child may be more motivated to work on breathing if he understands that a strong breathing pattern can help him project his voice when he needs to.

In therapy, you may want to teach a better respiratory pattern as part of the approach to vocal hygiene. You may also work to improve respiration as part of your overall approach to the child's hyperfunctional vocal pattern. Additionally, you might teach a better respiratory pattern to address a specific problem.

Some common problems that children may exhibit with respiration include:

- Forgetting to take a breath before they begin to talk
- Forgetting to take a breath at pauses during their speech
- Continuing to talk on low air when they should take another breath

The goals and treatment objectives to eliminate misuse of respiration and to teach appropriate use of respiratory support for speech and singing are:

Short-term Goal

Child will eliminate misuse of respiration and will use adequate respiratory support. (MU-R)

Treatment Objectives

1. Child will demonstrate understanding of difference in diaphragmatic and clavicular (or other abnormal patterns) breathing. (MU-R-1)
   a. when modeled by SLP (MU-R-1a)
   b. when the child imitates the patterns (MU-R-1b)

2. Child will use diaphragmatic breathing in supine on: (MU-R-2)
   a. simple exhalations (MU-R-2a)
   b. production of vowel sounds (MU-R-2b)
   c. imitation of phrases and sentences (MU-R-2c)

---

3. Child will use diaphragmatic breathing when standing on: (MU-R-3)
   a. simple exhalations (MU-R-3a)
   b. production of vowel sounds (MU-R-3b)
   c. imitation of phrases and sentences (MU-R-3c)

4. Child will use diaphragmatic breathing when sitting on: (MU-R-4)
   a. simple exhalations (MU-R-4a)
   b. production of vowel sounds (MU-R-4b)
   c. imitation of phrases and sentences (MU-R-4c)

5. Child will remember to take an adequate breath before beginning to speak in: (MU-R-5)
   a. short answers (MU-R-5a)
   b. reading passages (MU-R-5b)
   c. monologues (MU-R-5c)
   d. conversations (MU-R-5d)

6. Child will avoid speaking on low air by pausing for a breath during: (MU-R-6)
   a. reading passages (MU-R-6a)
   b. monologues (MU-R-6b)
   c. conversations (MU-R-6c)

Explaining respiration to the child

Chapter 4, pages 43-44, provides some suggestions on ways to explain the respiratory system to the child. Use of props like a balloon may help the child visualize what is happening when air is inhaled and exhaled. Help the child understand what this looks like and feels like as you demonstrate it and as the child performs the same movements.

MU-R Treatment Objective 1	Child will demonstrate understanding of difference in diaphragmatic and clavicular (or other abnormal patterns) breathing.

Demonstrating inappropriate and appropriate patterns

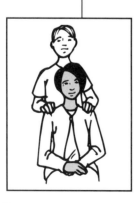

The easiest way to demonstrate to the child an inappropriate pattern, such as clavicular breathing, is to sit in a chair or stand so that the child can easily see the rise and fall of your shoulders. Exaggerate upward movement of the shoulders and upper chest as you breathe in and a falling motion as you exhale. While you're sitting in a chair, have the child stand behind you and place his hands on your shoulders. Then he will be able to feel the exaggerated rise and fall of the shoulders as you breathe.

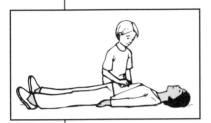

To demonstrate the correct pattern of breathing, lie in a supine position. Place your hand on your abdomen and the child's hand on top of yours. As you breathe in, make sure that your abdominal wall rises toward the ceiling and then falls back as you breathe out. Remind the child that the muscle called the *diaphragm* is what is helping you breathe, but that you cannot feel the diaphragm. Use the diagram on page 54 as needed to help the child understand the relationship between the diaphragm and the abdominal cavity. Be sure you have practiced this pattern before you demonstrate to the child. Point out to the child that your shoulders do not move as you breathe in.

Once the child understands how the abdominal cavity moves while you're in the supine position, demonstrate the pattern in the standing position. The child may continue to need some tactile feedback to help decide if your abdominal wall is moving.

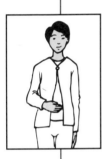

After you have demonstrated the correct and incorrect patterns of breathing to the child, the child needs to demonstrate that he understands the difference. Ask the child to be the judge and decide whether you are breathing correctly or incorrectly. From a standing position, demonstrate either an incorrect pattern with excessive movement of the shoulders or a correct pattern with good diaphragmatic breathing. You may have to exaggerate the diaphragmatic movement so the child can see movement of the abdominal wall. If the child is having difficulty, place his hands on your shoulders to feel shallow breathing or his hands on top of yours on your abdomen to feel diaphragmatic breathing.

Child imitates the patterns

MU-R Treatment Objective 2	Child will use diaphragmatic breathing in supine on: a. simple exhalations b. production of vowel sounds c. imitation of phrases and sentences
MU-R Treatment Objective 3	Child will use diaphragmatic breathing when standing on: a. simple exhalations b. production of vowel sounds c. imitation of phrases and sentences
MU-R Treatment Objective 4	Child will use diaphragmatic breathing when sitting on: a. simple exhalations b. production of vowel sounds c. imitation of phrases and sentences

When the child achieves a level of accuracy in discriminating between these two patterns, ask the child to imitate the patterns with you. You may want the child to lie on his back while he tries the diaphragmatic breathing. If the child is having difficulty making his abdomen move, place a book on his abdomen. It may be easier for the child to see the book rise and fall. The book should not touch the rib cage as it will move more easily if placed directly over the abdominal wall. Tell the child to make the book move up as he breathes in and let it fall down slowly as he blows out. The child may start by actually pushing out his stomach. That is fine, as the lungs will almost naturally fill with air as the thoracic cavity expands. Some children respond to the phrase "lead with your stomach."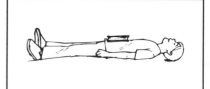

Have the child practice the incorrect pattern too to help him become more aware of his breathing pattern. This is called *negative practice*. You can both stand in front of a mirror to observe the rise and fall of the shoulders as he imitates the incorrect pattern.

Practicing diaphragmatic breathing

The child will need many practice activities in order to establish this new pattern of breathing. Appendix 7A, page 108, can be used as a handout so the child can practice this breathing pattern at home.

Begin with the child in a supine position, and have the child practice the pattern first by simply exhaling through closed lips, then making a vowel sound while exhaling. Coach the child to breathe in through his nose and blow out through his mouth. Make sure the child understands that he should not take a giant breath. Explain to the child that when we are talking or singing, we generally take a short breath (two seconds). If the child takes in too large an inhalation, it will be harder to control the exhalation. Count aloud as the child breathes in through his nose ("one, two") and as the child blows slowly out through his mouth. The child should be able to exhale to at least a count of five or six. If the child is having trouble controlling the speed of exhalation, have him produce a voiceless sibilant like "s" or "f." Producing a sibilant slows the exhalation. The child should be able to sustain that sound for 12-20 seconds.

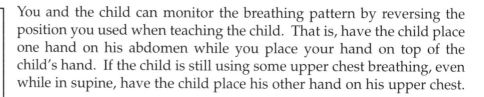

You and the child can monitor the breathing pattern by reversing the position you used when teaching the child. That is, have the child place one hand on his abdomen while you place your hand on top of the child's hand. If the child is still using some upper chest breathing, even while in supine, have the child place his other hand on his upper chest.

After the child has mastered production of vowel sounds on a slow exhalation, progress to using the new pattern of breathing when imitating words, phrases, and sentences.

Appendix 7B, pages 109-111, contains words, phrases, and sentences of increasing length, ranging from 2 syllables to 20 syllables. Depending on the respiratory capacity, the child may or may not be able to do sentences containing 20 syllables on one breath. This ability is also somewhat dependent on the child's age. Progress to a level where the child is producing an utterance that takes up most of the exhalation but does not require the child to speak on low air.

Once the child has mastered this pattern in supine, have him transfer the skill to a standing position, and then a sitting position. The sitting position is probably the most challenging because it is difficult to feel the abdominal wall moving while seated. The child can be encouraged to continue to place his hand on his abdominal wall in both

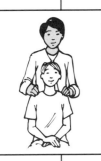

standing and sitting positions. The child may need to begin again with simply blowing air through the lips, and then progressing to vowel sounds. Some children may be able to skip those steps and proceed directly to imitating phrases and sentences while standing or sitting. If the child reverts to the pattern of excessive shoulder and upper chest movement while sitting or standing, place your hands on his shoulders and give downward pressure to discourage this movement.

Breathing Correctly During Speech Tasks

The next two goals address problems the child may have in managing breathing during conversation. The child may not take an adequate breath before he starts to talk, or he may forget to pause and take a breath during a long utterance and thus may continue talking long after he should have stopped for a new breath. These problems are very inter-related and sometimes hard to distinguish. In fact, it may not be necessary to distinguish between two separate goals for every child. Select one or both goals to get the point across to the child that he needs to slow down and breathe—either before or during an utterance.

MU-R Treatment Objective 5	Child will remember to take an adequate breath before beginning to speak in: a. short answers b. reading passages c. monologues d. conversations

MU-R Treatment Objective 6	Child will avoid speaking on low air by pausing for a breath during: a. reading passages b. monologues c. conversations

Short Answers

You can address these two treatment objectives in a hierarchy of tasks. When teaching the child to remember to take a breath before starting to talk, use an activity where you ask the child questions that require short answers. Some practice questions are provided in Appendix 7C, page 112. You can also use one of the characters in Appendix 7D (page 113) to signal the child to breathe.

Reading Passages

(Note: It is not likely that the child will speak on low air when providing a short answer so the hierarchy of activities for Treatment Objective 6 begins with reading passages, continues through monologues, and then into conversations.)

The value of using reading passages to teach the child when to take a breath is that you can mark on the passage where an appropriate place would be to pause for a breath. If the child is fairly young, it is likely that the level of the material he is reading will be comprised mostly of short sentences. If that is the case, you will simply need to remind the child to stop and take a breath at the end of each sentence. You should have a good idea of the number of syllables the child is able to produce on a single breath from the activities in Appendix 7B (pages 109-111) in which the child repeats words, phrases, and sentences of increasing length. Use these results as a guide to determine if you will need to mark pauses within a sentence in the reading material. Older children will certainly be reading material with longer sentences. Use a pen with colored ink or a highlighter to mark logical places to pause. Depending on the age of the child, you might have him help you decide where to pause. First mark all of the periods and commas. Then look for other logical places to pause.

Sample of pauses marked for student who can easily use 8-10 syllables/breath group

Ellen's team was going to be / the first one to give their oral report / in social studies./ Ellen, Jack, and Marianne / were partners on the project / and had been partners / on many projects before./ Because they had worked together / so many times before, / they had learned how to be a good team./ Anna's job, / besides being the one / who would actually / give most of the oral report, / was outlining the project / before they started./ Jack was the best researcher on the team, / partly because his aunt / was the school librarian./ Marianne was the best writer, / and she always volunteered / to be the team member / to complete the final draft.

Monologues

Once the child gets the idea about taking a breath at the beginning of an utterance and using pauses throughout reading passages, it is time to help the child practice using these skills in spontaneous speech. The child will not have any visual cues similar to the slash marks used in the reading passage. You can use one of the characters from Appendix 7D as a visual reminder to take a breath.

Give the child a topic and explain that you want him to talk about that topic for about one minute. You may have to model how to produce a monologue, as many children are uncomfortable with this task at first. Tell the child that you want him to remember to take a breath before each sentence and to stop and pause for breath before he feels that he is running out of air. You can hold up the character as needed throughout the monologue to cue him to take a breath. A list of possible topics that could be used for the monologues is provided in Appendix 7E, page 114. If the child has trouble with monologues, you can begin the task by using the stimulus items in Appendix 7F, page 115, that require the child to list things as his answer. This task will usually elicit pauses as it is natural to stop between items as you list them.

Conversations

You can use the same list of topics in Appendix 7E to have a conversation with the child. Conversations may be an easier situation for the child to remember to breathe if short answers are required throughout the conversation. When you take your turn, it is a logical place for the child to take a breath. You may have to pay closer attention in this activity to make sure the child is taking a breath before he starts to talk.

Using Negative Practice

If the child is having a hard time "feeling" what you mean by talking on low air, try the following activity. Have the child blow out all his air and not take in a new breath. Then have him count as far as he can without taking another breath. Ask the child to note how this feels. Does he feel tightness in his throat? In his chest and abdomen? Does his voice sound more strained? Then have the child take a good breath and try counting again, using pauses as you signal him. Ask him to note any differences he feels. There should be less tension and no straining to say the numbers.

Relaxing the Muscles

If the child seems very tight, you can teach a relaxation exercise that might help him use a better breathing pattern. Have the child stand up and lean over with his head and arms hanging down. He should be loose, like a rag doll. Make sure the child is not holding his head up or his neck rigid.

Have the child take a breath and as he exhales, have him slowly come up, inch by inch. It may help the child for you to touch his lower back, then his middle back, then his shoulders, and then his head to indicate the order in which you want him to come out of the "rag doll" position. Remind the child that the last thing to come up will be his head.

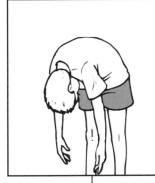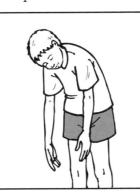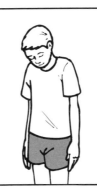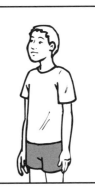

Summary

Respiration is one of the foundations on which good vocal quality is built. Spending time teaching the child how to achieve good breath support for speech and singing will make it easier for the child to complete many of the tasks to improve phonation and resonance/focus. Respiration activities are easy for the child to practice at home and can easily be practiced in other situations, such as riding in the car or when listening in class.

Breathing Practice

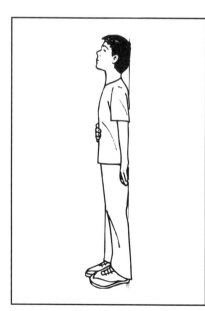

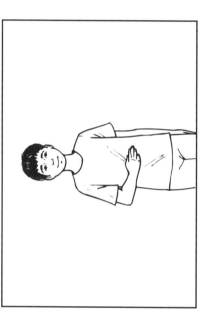

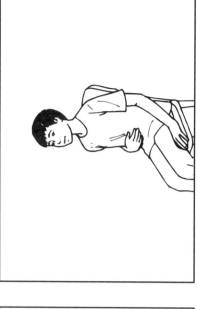

Lie on your back.
Place your hand on your abdomen below
   your belly button.
Feel your "stomach" go up as you breathe in.
Feel your "stomach" fall as you breathe out.
You can slow down your breathing out by
   saying "s" or "f."

Stand in front of a mirror.
Place your hand on your abdomen.
Feel your "stomach" go out as you breathe in.
Feel your "stomach" go in as you breathe out.
You can slow down your breathing out by
   saying "s" or "f."

Sit in a chair in front of a mirror.
Place your hand on your abdomen.
Feel your "stomach" go out as you breathe in.
Feel your "stomach" go in as you breathe out.
You can slow down your breathing out by
   saying "s" or "f."

After you have practiced the breathing several times, try saying a vowel sound when the air comes out:

   ahh   ooo   eeee   uhhh

Then have someone read _____ words, phrases, or sentences from pages 109-111 to you one at a time. Repeat each
                      (number)

phrase as you breathe out. You are working on words, phrases, and sentences that have _____ syllables. Try to practice

_____ times a day.

Utterances of Increasing Lengths

Two Syllables

apple
open
okay
inside
outside
upstairs
homework
cat food
cupcake
baseball

Three Syllables

not in here
Way to go.
I love dogs.
cold water
telephone
Kick the can.
Go to bed.
Answer me.
envelope
Do not sing.

Four Syllables

Let's go outside.
Help me up, please.
It's time to go.
Read me a book.
Mountains are high.
John Smith lives here.
yellow daisies
Wake up happy.
Children like toys.
The sky is blue.

Five Syllables

Where is the new dog?
Can you see Pedro?
Enjoy the movie.
Open the window.
Welcome to the club.
Enter carefully.
Empty the bottle.
Run as fast as Joe.
Lemonade is good.
Nothing works better.

Six Syllables

I'm not ready for that.
My cat is very fat.
Her hair is not too long.
Please copy the letter.
My sweater is purple.
January is cold.
Next month is November.
because I want you to
Aunt Maria made those.
Computer games are fun.

Seven Syllables

The dogs are making a mess.
Bob decided to go home.
Amanda is amazing.
Any time you are ready.
Stephanie likes bananas.
natural peanut butter
Kittens like to play outside.
Adam likes baseball better.
The telephone rang a lot.
German is a hard language.

Eight Syllables

I don't know where my homework is.
Basketball is Susan's best sport.
Pink is the color of my room.
Candy canes are red and white striped.
Matthew sleeps with a firm pillow.
Alabama is a big state.
Geese fly south in the winter months.
Being very late is not good.
The phone book has lots of pages.
The calculator does not work.

Nine Syllables

Kentucky has a lot of horses.
The teacher told us to listen now.
I think cats are much smarter than dogs.
My watermelon was very good.
Jennifer did not complete her work.
coconuts, apples, and pineapples
Football is a long and boring game.
Butterflies are seen in the spring time.
My brother's old middle school is gone.
My red pants are at the dry cleaners.

10 Syllables

Can you believe it is time to go home?
The Wildcats have won a lot of their games.
The best book I've read is Harry Potter.
The turtle walked slowly around the pond.
Repeat the numbers from the beginning.
The plastic dinosaur fell off the chair.
Lexington used to be a small city.
Would you believe that it is the new year?
Lemons are yellow and they taste bitter.
Do you want to see a movie tonight?

11 Syllables

The baseball team is practicing tomorrow.
I'd rather read a book than watch a movie.
Did your new bicycle arrive yesterday?
List problems you have had or think you will have.
The airplane may be late but we will make it.
What will you do on your very next birthday?
I can't believe I have finished this project.
The basketball team ran around the court twice.
Would you rather eat spaghetti and meatballs?
I made a wish when I blew out the candles.

12 Syllables

My big sister is going to college next year.
The boys ate pickles and peanut butter for lunch.
Someone said that our math teacher lives on a boat.
The baby was born on Saturday afternoon.
The moonlight was not bright enough to light the sky.
The mice in June's bathroom were not very scary.
The leaves will turn red, gold, and yellow in autumn.
The recycled paper is made up of old trees.
I will be ready to go home at five o'clock.
That horse did not want to eat any more carrots.

13 Syllables

You will now begin seeing the tutor on Mondays.
The animals that I like best of all are tigers.
The lunch will begin at noon and end at three thirty.
Nothing can smell worse than my two brothers' undershirts.
Elephants are enormous and have gigantic toes.
We will need an instructor to lead the orchestra.
The teachers like to point out interesting findings.
The Knoxville Zoo contained eleven baby monkeys.
The twelve-year-old girl took a class on baby-sitting.
Never tell your teacher that the homework is stupid.

14 Syllables

Life was okay until my father found the large, gray box.
The mysterious message was left by the old mummy.
Balancing between school and sports is very difficult.
Telephone conversations typically last two minutes.
Nina enjoys spending her summers in New Mexico.
The Appalachian Mountains are really spectacular.
New York City is a fun place to shop and have dinner.
Callie's younger brother ate too much fish on vacation.
Friday is always the best day of the week for José.
Suzanne and Kari went skating at the birthday party.

15 Syllables

Fairy tales only exist in a child's imagination.
You are about to enter the Museum of Ancient Times.
Steven is reading "The Indian in the Cupboard" at school.
Hawaii is home to pretty flowers and lots of surfers.
Carlos told me that junk food is not good for a growing boy.
If you are lost, you should try to find a police officer
Exercising will help you feel much stronger and grow strong bones.
Whenever Jai Lin has some time, she gets on the Internet.
Brownies and milk are Shonita's number one after-school snack.
I walked past Elizabeth and found a seat near the front row.

16 Syllables

You and your class are going on a field trip to the museum.
It will cost each student forty dollars to join the science club.
When we get to Jessica's house, we'll give each other a high five.
A student must listen carefully in order to get good grades.
My little brother likes to lock himself in the bathroom to hide.
Grandma Linda enjoys reading the newspaper in her spare time.
Stories about David reveal his unusual pets and his magical powers.
The exact distance that a worm can jump has never been measured.
Can you imagine a plant that only blooms once each century?
Captain Alexander ordered the cannons to be fired at sea.

17 Syllables

Mindy ate twenty candy bars and had a stomachache for two days.
Caterpillars build cocoons before they become pretty butterflies.
Tulips are bright and beautiful and many people like to grow them.
The making of a dictionary is a slow and tedious job.
More than 2000 men and women were killed in the big Johnstown flood.
Yellow fever is a well-known disease carried by most mosquitoes.
For almost 5000 years, cats have been kept as pets in many homes.
When I was a little girl, Kim was my baby-sitter on Fridays.
"The upstairs bathroom needs to be cleaned immediately," said my mom.
If the children are very bad, they do not get to select stickers.

18 Syllables

I reread the chapter several times and still do not understand it.
Tim understood that the only way to win would be to try extra hard.
Hollywood bought Melinda's story and made it a successful movie.
A bad thunderstorm in the desert can bring unexpected surprises.
Each day, the guards carefully protect the king, the queen, and all the children.
From earliest times, humans have looked to the sky and wished to fly like birds.
The fourth graders seemed to like the slippery slide on the playground the best.
My mother and father like to watch "Wheel of Fortune" on TV each night.
The large African Rock Python lives in the savannas of Africa.
Computers are becoming lighter, faster, and less expensive each year.

19 Syllables

Apples and bananas are the best kind of fruit to eat during the summer.
English has become a universal language in many other countries.
Spaghetti and meatballs are a good meal to have when lots of friends come over.
We all dream but can never recall our dreams when we wake up in the morning.
In the early 1800s, people were fascinated with sap from trees.
Jordan walked home from school sadly because his mother forgot to pick him up.
Tiffany watched as the creepy spiders crawled up the walls of the big, red barn.
Leona likes to eat peanut butter and pickle sandwiches for dinner.
Terry wished to have an elephant and acrobat at his birthday party.
Dalmatian dogs are very active and like to run outside in the summer.

20 Syllables

When you go to the air and space museum, get a map so you can find your way.
I went into the kitchen and Nancy said, "Where have you been? Why didn't you call?"
All night I dream about bars on my window and guards standing beside the front door.
Bats are not as scary as you think; they only need one teaspoon of blood a day.
The Depression that followed the stock market crash saw lots of people without jobs.
Fortune hunters used to think if they found an elephants' graveyard, they would be rich.
Jigsaw puzzles generally became available in the 1900s.
Whales breathe heavily through their blowholes, flies taste with their feet, and snakes have no eyelids.
Anthony likes to go fishing in rivers but only when it is not raining.
The angry grizzly bear madly opened the van door and ate all of our good food.

Questions to Elicit Short Answers

1. How do cats take a bath?
2. How do children learn to swim?
3. How does a giraffe eat leaves from a tree?
4. How do you make a sandwich?
5. What are windows used for?
6. What can grow in a garden?
7. What can you do in the snow?
8. What do people do at football games?
9. What do people do at the beach?
10. What do people do with a telephone?
11. What do you do when you catch a cold?
12. What do you like about computers?
13. What do you wish for on your birthday?
14. What happens to trees in the fall?
15. What happens to your voice when you yell?
16. What would you do if you found a ten-dollar bill?
17. Where can you go on a bus?
18. Where does the sun go when it's dark?
19. Who lives with you?
20. Why are you coming to see me?
21. Why can't we see the stars every night?
22. Why do dogs bark?
23. Why do elephants have a trunk?
24. Why do men shave?
25. Why do people wear eyeglasses?
26. Why do people wear shoes?
27. Why do people wear watches?
28. Why do teachers give homework?
29. Why do teachers write on the board?
30. Why is summer the best time of year?

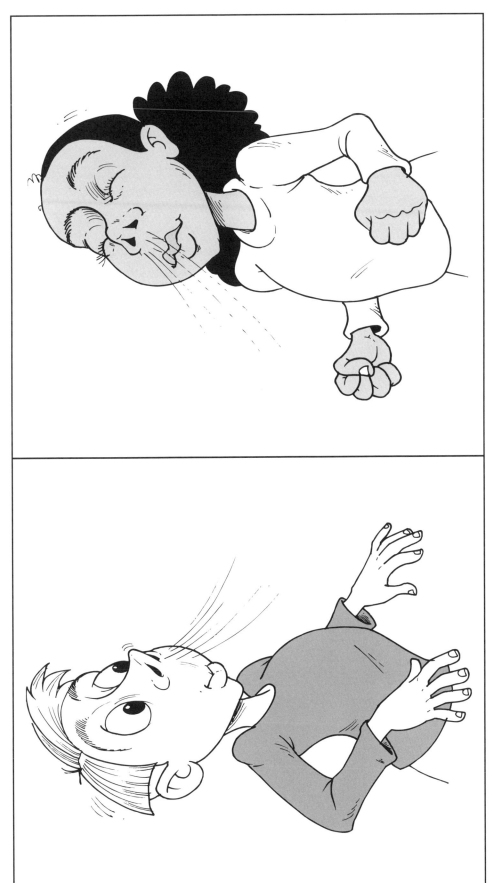

Take-a-Breath Timmy

Take-a-Breath Tammy

Appendix 7D
The Source for Children's Voice Disorders

Topics for Monologues and Conversations

Tell me everything you can about:

a circus	ghosts
a playground	grandparents
a library	hiking
airplanes	horses
babies	islands
baseball	money
birds	mountains
birthday parties	musical instruments
board games	oceans
boats	outer space
brothers	playing cards
bugs	restaurants
cars	school
cats	sisters
computers	snakes
cowboys	soccer
dentists	swimming
desserts	teachers
doctors	toys
dogs	trains
farm animals	weddings
football	weekends
fruits	zoos

Ways to Elicit List Responses

Who lives in a zoo?
What kinds of animals live on a farm?
What is in a closet?
What can be found in a shopping center?
What can you buy at a bakery?
What can you buy at a drugstore?
What are popular desserts?
What do you like to watch on TV?
If we were creating a new classroom, what things would we need to put in it?
If you were creating a new playground, what things would you want to put in it?

Name animals that live in the ocean.
Name different flavors of ice cream.
Name different sports played in the Olympics.
Name different streets in your neighborhood.
Name some Presidents of the United States.
Name some things you can grow in a garden.
Name the colors in the rainbow.
Name the other students in your class.
Name ways you can travel.
Name different kinds of birds.

Tell me all the things you need to pack in a suitcase for a long trip.
Tell me all the things you can think of that can go on a pizza.
Tell me some costumes children wear on Halloween.
Tell me some things I could find in your refrigerator.
Tell me some things I could find in your cubby/desk.
Tell me the names of people in your family.
Tell me what you like about school.
Tell me some of your favorite toys.
Tell me some things a teacher has on his/her desk.
Tell me some things a coach would have in his/her office.

8 | Treatment for Phonation

You might expect the chapter on phonation in a book on voice disorders to appear earlier in the sequence of chapters about treatment. However, there are many aspects of voice disorders other than the use of the vocal folds for phonation. It is difficult to compartmentalize all of the physiological components that contribute to a pleasant sounding, healthy voice. So, although this chapter focuses on techniques for treating problems with phonation, it will also draw on information from other treatment chapters.

This chapter addresses three aspects of phonation that may be problematic for children with voice disorders:

- Volume (loudness)
- Pitch
- Onset

These three aspects of phonation often interact. For example, when the child is asked to elevate pitch, she often elevates loudness as well. When the child is asked to lower volume, she may inadvertently develop too breathy of an initiation for her phonation. Despite these limitations, the information in this chapter is broken down according to these three major categories of volume, pitch, and onset.

The goals and treatment objectives to eliminate misuse of phonation and to teach appropriate use of the laryngeal mechanism for speech are:

Short-term Goal 1

Child will eliminate misuse of phonation characterized by inappropriate volume and will use loudness appropriate to the situation. (MU-P-V)

Treatment Objectives

1. Child will discriminate between three vocal loudness levels modeled by SLP. (MU-P-V-1)

2. Child will produce each of the three loudness levels in: (MU-P-V-2)
   a. words and short phrases (MU-P-V-2a)
   b. sentences (MU-P-V-2b)
   c. conversation (MU-P-V-2c)

3. Child will select and use the appropriate loudness level in a variety of situations. (MU-P-V-3)

Short-term Goal 2

Child will eliminate misuse of phonation characterized by inappropriate pitch and will use optimal pitch in all situations. (MU-P-P)

Treatment Objectives

1. Child will discriminate between low and high pitches modeled by SLP. (MU-P-P-1)

2. Child will discriminate between inappropriate and target pitch in audiotape/live samples of own speech. (MU-P-P-2)

continued on next page

---

3. Child will consistently use target pitch (optimal fundamental frequency) in: (MU-P-P-3)
    a. words and short phrases (MU-P-P-3a)
    b. sentences (MU-P-P-3b)
    c. conversation (MU-P-P-3c)

Short-term Goal 3

Child will eliminate misuse of phonation characterized by inappropriate onset and will exhibit appropriate vocal quality/easy onset. (MU-P-O)

Treatment Objectives

1. Child will discriminate between breathy, hard attack and adequate onset of phonation modeled by SLP. (MU-P-O-1)

2. Child will discriminate between breathy, hard attack and adequate onset in audiotape/live sample of own phonation. (MU-P-O-2)

3. Child will produce appropriate/easy onset in/on: (MU-P-O-3)
    a. vowels (MU-P-O-3a)
    b. vowel-initiated words and phrases (MU-P-O-3b)
    c. words and phrases beginning with consonants (MU-P-O-3c)
    d. sentences (MU-P-O-3d)
    e. conversation (MU-P-O-3e)

Explaining How Phonation Occurs

Chapter 4 contains information about how to talk with the child about the vocal mechanism. Obviously a child is not going to understand something as complex as the aerodynamic-myoelastic theory (Van den Berg 1958) or the flow-induced self-oscillating system (Titze 1988). If you show the child a picture of the larynx and how the position of the vocal folds changes from open during breathing to closed during phonation, it will help the child understand the muscular movement that approximates the vocal folds. However, it's also important for the child to understand the relationship between respiration and phonation and the important role that air from the lungs plays in moving/vibrating the vocal folds. A cube of Jell-O makes a nice model for demonstrating a quick vibratory movement. As you smack the Jell-O with a spoon, explain to the child that air from the lungs makes the vocal folds vibrate in ways similar to the jiggly Jell-O movement.

Volume Problems

Talking too loudly is a common problem in children with vocal abuse. The child may be unaware that her volume is inappropriate to the situation. In fact, she may not be able to discriminate when she is talking too loudly from when she is using an appropriate volume. Explain to the child that the appropriate way to increase volume is to use more forceful exhalation of air from the lungs. Tell the child that sometimes we forget and use the muscles in our throat to force out the louder volume. If the child is having a hard time understanding this concept, you might use activities from Chapter 7, pages 102-106.

Understanding different loudness levels

MU-P-V Treatment Objective 1	Child will discriminate between three vocal loudness levels modeled by SLP.

It's not enough to tell the child that she is talking too loudly. The child will find herself in different situations that require different loudness levels. For very young children, you may need to use only two loudness distinctions: inside voice and outside voice. However, most school-age children should be able to understand, discriminate, and produce three different loudness levels: quiet library voice, medium classroom voice, and loud playground voice. The descriptors *quiet*, *medium*, and *loud* have been added to these terms purposefully. If we used the environmental labels only (library, classroom, playground), the child might be confused. We're going to teach that the medium level of loudness is called a *classroom voice*, but there are times that the quiet library voice and even the loud playground voice might be appropriate in the classroom.

If these labels are not meaningful for the child, you can also use animal labels (e.g., mouse, cat, tiger). You can explain that if these animals could talk, their voices would probably match their sizes. That is, a mouse would have a quiet voice, a cat would have a medium voice, and tiger would have a loud voice. (See Appendix 8A, page 126, for pictures to help cue the child.)

Library voice (or mouse voice)

The most important characteristic for the child to understand about a quiet voice is that you do not mean a whisper. Demonstrate the difference between a whisper and a quiet voice that you would use in a library. Explain to the child that producing a whisper takes a lot of muscle tension and is hard on the voice, not easy on the voice.

Other analogies that you might use to describe this very quiet volume might include the voice you would use in the back seat of the car when you do not want your mom to hear what you're saying, a voice you would use in a fancy restaurant, or a voice you would use at practice after the coach has said "no more talking."

Classroom voice (or cat voice)

This level of volume is the one typically used in one-on-one situations. It is the voice the child would use to answer the teacher's question in a presumably quiet classroom environment. This is the loudness level that the child should be using the majority of the time.

Playground voice (or tiger voice)

When describing and modeling what a playground voice might sound like, stress that you do not mean yelling or screaming. A playground voice is the voice that is slightly louder than the average volume. It is the voice you would have to use if talking over noise (e.g., talking to the person next to you at a basketball game, gaining the teacher's attention when there is a lot of noise in the classroom, talking to someone in another room at home).

You can also provide examples of times a child might need to use her voice at this volume in order to project the sound. This might include giving a speech in a classroom or participating in a play on a stage. When you are demonstrating this louder voice, reinforce that you are producing a loud voice by using increased air pressure from the lungs. A good way to show the child what you mean is to have the child stand up, take in a good breath, and say "ah" at her quiet level. Have her hold the sound. Give a quick push to the abdomen to force air up. You and the child will hear a change in loudness.

Discriminating the three levels

Once the child seems to understand the three different loudness levels, provide the child with some practice to see if she can reliably discriminate which loudness level you are using. You can use the pictures in Appendix 8A (page 126) in a variety of ways for this activity. You can model loudness levels and have the child point to the picture that matches each production. You can also have the child hold up one of the pictures. Then you produce a loudness level that may or may not match the picture. The child tells if your production was appropriate.

Practicing loudness levels

MU-P-V Treatment Objective 2	Child will produce each of the three loudness levels in: a. words and short phrases b. sentence level utterances c. conversation

After the child has demonstrated accuracy in discriminating among the three loudness levels, provide practice for the child in using the different levels. Start with producing the levels in short utterances and progress to maintaining them during short conversations. Again, you can use the pictures in Appendix 8A for this practice. Place one of the pictures on the table and tell the child that until you change the picture, you will each use that loudness level as you talk. Engage the child in speech activities that require a word or short phrase answer, sentence level utterance, or conversation. Any board game that requires taking turns provides an excellent opportunity for practicing loudness levels.

Maintaining appropriate loudness levels

MU-P-V Treatment Objective 3	Child will select and use the appropriate loudness level in a variety of situations.

The real hurdle is having the child use the appropriate loudness levels in real-life situations. To be successful may require the use of a specific behavioral management program and help from adults throughout the day. (See Chapter 4, pages 45-47, for more information on implementing a behavior change program.)

You can practice maintaining appropriate loudness levels by using Appendix 8B, page 127. These pictures show a variety of situations a child might encounter. Have the child match each picture to the appropriate loudness level using the library, classroom, and playground pictures in Appendix 8A. There may be more than one appropriate loudness level to use in each situation. For example, the child might indicate that a library voice is needed in the classroom when the students are working in small groups but the playground voice may be needed when trying to gain the teacher's attention. There are no absolute answers as long as the child can demonstrate appropriate loudness at the level she has chosen and tell why she selected that level.

Some of the situations depicted are those the child may have been asked to avoid (e.g., child is in one room talking to someone in a different room). Take advantage of the opportunity to reinforce that rule when you discuss that picture.

After practicing appropriate loudness for a variety of situations, it is time for the child to start applying the skills in day-to-day life. The child can record the times she practices monitoring her loudness using Appendix 8C, page 128. Typically the target will be getting the child to use the medium loudness level rather than a playground voice. You will need to find some adults or older children (perhaps a sibling or a student from a higher grade) to serve as coaches for the child. They can help remind her to use the appropriate loudness level in various day-to-day situations. Let each "coach" know what the target is and explain how you would like the coach to help.

A good nonverbal signal for a coach to use to indicate when the student is talking too loudly is to pull gently on his ear. This cue signals the child to lower her volume. Some children respond to pictures in the problem situations. The classroom teacher might post a picture of the desired loudness level on the board or tape it to the child's desk to help her remember. The librarian might have a picture of the "mouse" voice in the library (although many librarians already have signs reminding students to be quiet). If the child is a tactile learner, she could carry a special reminder in her pocket (e.g., three small stones of differing sizes to represent the three loudness levels). The child could carry all three, or just the one that is the target volume size.

To achieve carryover at home, it is helpful if the child's parents and siblings are willing and able to model appropriate loudness. You'll need to make sure that these family members are aware of the different levels and the terminology you use to describe each one.

Pitch Problems

The goals and treatment objectives to work on pitch reflect that the child may be using too low or too high a pitch. The approaches shared in this chapter do not require the use of instrumentation to change pitch. The child should have undergone an instrumental evaluation of voice that would indicate if her pitch is too high or too low and if pitch is the primary problem. Pitch problems are not typical in pre-adolescent children. Often if the pitch is perceived as too low or too high, it may be that the child is trying to compensate for another problem (e.g., the child's voice keeps cracking at one pitch, so he tries a different pitch to sound clearer) or that the pitch change is secondary to an organic problem (e.g., a child with nodules may have a pitch that sounds lower because of the added bulk on the vocal folds).

In either case, what really needs to be treated is the underlying reason for the change in pitch. For example, if hyperfunctional use of the mechanism has caused inflammation of the vocal folds and subsequently a lower pitch, then techniques to improve hyperfunction should be used. If vocally abusive behaviors have made the child sound hoarse and low-pitched, then the vocal abuses should be addressed. When the laryngeal mechanism is healthier, the child's voice should sound better without direct work on the pitch.

Sometimes what is perceived as too high a pitch is really a resonance problem. That is, the child has her voice focused too far in the front of her mouth and the resulting quality is thin and high. (See Chapter 9, pages 137-146, for more information.) If that's the case, using resonance techniques to refocus the voice will result in an appropriate sounding pitch.

Several reasons that a child might actually have an inappropriate pitch as the primary problem might be (Stemple et al. 2000):

- emotional problems—if the child is depressed, the pitch may be low
- fatigue—if the child is tired, she is likely to use poor breath support and drop the pitch to a lower level
- talking too loudly—when a louder intensity is used, pitch increases as well

If the child truly is using too high or too low a pitch as the primary problem, then the techniques listed below can be used.

> *Note: This goal should be selected sparingly and with a clear understanding that inappropriate pitch is the primary problem and not a secondary symptom. Training the child to use a pitch that is too low or too high may actually harm the larynx.*
>
> ### Short-term Goal
>
> Child will eliminate misuse of phonation characterized by inappropriate pitch and will use optimal pitch in all situations. (MU-P-P)
>
> ### Treatment Objectives
>
> 1. Child will discriminate between low and high pitches modeled by SLP. (MU-P-P-1)
>
> 2. Child will discriminate between inappropriate and target pitch in audiotape/live samples of own speech. (MU-P-P-2)
>
> 3. Child will consistently use target pitch (optimal fundamental frequency) in: (MU-P-P-3)
>
>   a. words and short phrases (MU-P-P-3a)
>
>   b. sentence level utterances (MU-P-P-3b)
>
>   c. conversation (MU-P-P-3c)

Discrimination of different pitches

MU-P-P Treatment Objective 1	Child will discriminate between low and high pitches modeled by SLP.

MU-P-P Treatment Objective 2	Child will discriminate between inappropriate and target pitch in audiotape/live samples of own speech.

The child needs to understand the difference in the concepts of *low* and *high* and be able to tell whether a particular voice is low or high. You can model voices that are high pitched and low pitched and/or use fictional and cartoon characters as examples of voices that are high and low. Pictures of characters to help you show this contrast can be found in Appendix 8D, page 129.

You can also play an audiotape sample of the child's speech and point out occurrences of pitch that is appropriate and pitch that is inappropriate (either too high or too low). The child will have one problem—a pitch that is too high or too low. If the child's pitch is too high, it will probably be too high all of the time. A child with pitch that is too low may exhibit pitch that is too low all of the time or just drop into a pitch that is too low at the end of an utterance. A child who drops the pitch too low at the end of an utterance may be using glottal fry. *Glottal fry* is the lowest register of the voice and sounds like a creaking door or sputtering motor (Boone et al. 2005). A child will not need help distinguishing high from low pitch in her own voice, but rather practice distinguishing appropriate pitch from the low pitch she is using or practice distinguishing appropriate pitch from the high pitch she is using.

The child also needs to become aware of when pitch is not appropriate while listening to live speech samples. Engage the child in activities that will elicit short utterances. See if the child can listen as she talks and indicate when her pitch is inappropriate. The characters in Appendix 8E, page 130, may help. If you're working with a child whose pitch is too high, use the picture of High Hank or High Hannah (depending on the gender of your client). If you're working with a child whose pitch is too low, use the picture of Low Lou or Low Louetta.

Learning how to make and use the target pitch

MU-P-P Treatment Objective 3	Child will consistently use target pitch (optimal fundamental frequency) in: a. words and short phrases b. sentences c. conversation

The first step in establishing the use of the new pitch is to make sure the child can produce the pitch after you model it. Start by using a vowel sound at the pitch you want the child to use and have her say the sound with you. Then have the child produce that vowel sound at the target pitch without a model. Tape record the sound once it is produced appropriately. Then have the child listen to the sound on the tape as you progress through longer utterances into conversation. To help the child understand what you mean by the target pitch, use a pitch pipe or a note on a musical instrument.

Once the child can consistently replicate the pitch of the extended vowel sound, move to the next step—having the child produce words that begin with a vowel sound at that same pitch. A list of words, phrases, and sentences beginning with vowel sounds can be found in Appendix 8F, page 131. Continue to increase the length of utterance and difficulty of the situations in which you expect the child to use the higher pitch. Appendix 8G, page 132, contains sentences that begin with vowel sounds. Utterances that begin with vowel sounds may be easier for the child than phrases or sentences that start with consonants. In order to keep the production at the appropriate pitch, the child may first need to produce the word, phrase, or sentence in a sing-song manner. To help the child transition to a more natural sounding form of speech, have the child hold the vowel sound at the target pitch to make sure she is starting at the right place and then finish the rest of the sentence in a more natural intonation.

Using negative practice

If the child is having a hard time maintaining the target pitch, have her practice some utterances at the inappropriate pitch. That is, have her repeat a sentence at the target pitch and then again at the inappropriate pitch. Ask her to note not only how these two *sound* different, but how they *feel* different. When the target pitch is used, there should be no strain on the mechanism. The child may also be able to "feel" the resonance of the utterance (See Chapter 9, page 143).

Voice Onset and Quality

Although there are many other aspects to quality, voice onset is a characteristic that is easier to explain, easier for children to understand, and easier to modify than, for example, telling the child not to use a voice that sounds so harsh. In addition, if the onset of the phrase is modified so that it is ideal, it is likely that the rest of the utterance will be produced with better quality. The two basic problems with onset are:

- Onset is too hard, called *hard glottal attack*
- Onset is too breathy (a much less common problem)

We will focus mostly on techniques to eliminate hard glottal attack since this is the more common problem and is harmful to the vocal mechanism. We'll provide some limited information on addressing a voice that is too breathy, the other extreme from a hard glottal attack.

The goals and objectives for improving the quality of onset include:

Short-term Goal

Child will eliminate misuse of phonation characterized by inappropriate onset and will exhibit appropriate vocal quality. (MU-P-O)

Treatment Objectives

1. Child will discriminate between breathy, hard attack and adequate onset of phonation modeled by the SLP. (MU-P-O-1)

2. Child will discriminate between breathy, hard attack and adequate onset in audiotape/live samples of own phonation. (MU-P-O-2)

3. Child will produce appropriate/easy onset on/in: (MU-P-O-3)
   a. vowels (MU-P-O-3a)
   b. vowel-initiated words and phrases (MU-P-O-3b)
   c. words and phrases beginning with consonants (MU-P-O-3c)
   d. sentences (MU-P-O-3d)
   e. conversation (MU-P-O-3e)

Discrimination of different onsets: hard, breathy, appropriate (easy)

MU-P-O Treatment Objective 1	Child will discriminate between breathy, hard attack, and adequate onset of phonation modeled by SLP.

MU-P-O Treatment Objective 2	Child will discriminate between breathy, hard attack and adequate onset in audiotape/live samples of own speech.

The child will have to understand the differences among the hard attack, extremely breathy onset, and appropriate (easy) onset. Because the use of a more breathy onset (e.g., words that start with "h") is used as a treatment to eliminate the hard attack, you may have to spend some time contrasting this with an onset that has too much air. You can model each type of onset or use examples of people the child knows (or has seen on TV or in the movies) who use these different types of onset. Some public speakers (e.g., preachers/ministers) use a very hard onset. Hard onset occurs when the speaker closes the glottis and builds up pressure below the vocal folds before producing the sound. It may occur only on the first word in the utterance or on each word. Use the characters in Appendix 8H, page 133, to represent different onsets.

You can also play an audiotape sample of the child's speech and point out occurrences of onset that are inappropriate (too hard or too breathy). The child will have either a hard attack or a breathy attack—but not both. A child will not need help distinguishing hard attack from breathy onset in her own voice, but rather practice distinguishing hard onset from easy onset or practice distinguishing breathy onset from easy onset.

The child also needs to become aware of what type of onset she is using in spontaneous speech. Engage the child in activities that will elicit short utterances. See if the child can listen as she talks and indicate when she hears a hard attack or a breathy onset. You may need to manipulate the stimuli to make it easier for the child to hear. Words and phrases beginning with vowel sounds make it easier to hear the onset of the word. (See Appendix 8F, page 131, and Appendix 8G, page 132.)

Learning to use easy onset

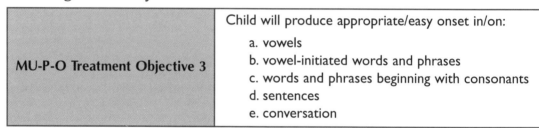

MU-P-O Treatment Objective 3	Child will produce appropriate/easy onset in/on: a. vowels b. vowel-initiated words and phrases c. words and phrases beginning with consonants d. sentences e. conversation

Whether the child is using the more common hard attack or is too breathy, the goal is to teach the child how to use easy onset. Easy onset involves a gentle approximation of the vocal folds at the beginning of the utterance. The exhaled air blows gently over the vocal folds and the phonation starts gently.

Using "h" words to demonstrate airflow

To help the child understand the concept of airflow moving past the vocal folds, have the child repeat some words that begin with the "h" sound (see Appendix 8I, page 134). Tell the child to let the air start to flow on the "h" and then produce the rest of the word with an easy sound.

Using easy onset in different contexts

After the child is able to produce the "h" words with good airflow, try words beginning with vowels. You can tell the child to imagine that there is an "h" in front of the word. For example, if the word is *air*, the child can pretend the word is *hair* and start some air coming out before she starts to say the vowel sound. The words in Appendix 8J, page 135, have word pairs. One word of each pair begins with a vowel and the other word rhymes and starts with "h" (e.g., *am/ham, art/heart*). You'll want to wean the child from using "h" as this is not truly an easy onset, but a breathy onset.

Other techniques to encourage easy onset of phonation

The *yawn-sigh* (Boone et al. 2005) is another technique that will help to eliminate the hard glottal attack. Explain to the child that a yawn helps the muscles in the mouth and throat open and relax. Have the child yawn several times and feel how the throat opens. Then ask the child to produce a very light sound on the exhalation after the yawn. When the child has mastered this task, have her say words that start with the "h" sound or an open vowel on the exhalation.

Another analogy that may help the child get the idea of easy onset is to talk about a radio. Ask the child to imagine that we have turned the radio on, but we have the volume down all the way. We gradually turn the volume up. Demonstrate as you say a word that starts with a vowel sound and you gradually increase the volume. That is what easy onset sounds like. In contrast, ask the child to think about the radio in the car. Maybe the volume was really loud when the car was turned off. The next time the car is started, the radio will blare loudly. Demonstrate as you use a hard attack on a vowel-initiated word. You can use the vowel words, phrases, and sentences in Appendix 8F, page 131, to help the child produce the easy onset.

As the child masters the strategy when saying vowels, gradually increase the complexity of the utterance to words and phrases (see Appendix 8G, page 132). The next step, words and phrases that start with consonants, may be difficult at first for the child. It is impossible to use an easy onset with some types of consonants (e.g., plosives). For these consonants, teach the child to produce the plosive and then use easy onset on the vowel following the plosive. Words that begin with other types of consonants (e.g., stridents, fricatives, affricates, nasals) are much easier to manage if the consonant is voiced. Teach the child to use an easy onset by slightly extending the consonant. If the consonant is voiceless, the child will need to apply the easy onset to the next vowel. Appendix 8K, page 136, has words and short sentences divided into stop consonants, voiceless continuants, and voiced continuants for practice.

Continue to help the child apply this new pattern of onset in longer sentences and finally in conversational speech. You may not totally eliminate the incorrect pattern. For example, you may still hear a hard onset when the child is excited. However, if the child is able to significantly reduce the occurrences of inappropriate onset, there should be a positive impact on overall vocal quality.

Using Instrumentation for Phonation Goals

If you have access to the *Kay Visi-Pitch* or *Sonaspeech*, they can be used to help the child understand the concepts of *loudness*, *pitch*, and *onset*. The instruments can be used throughout therapy to provide biofeedback to the child. If you don't have this type of instrumentation, you can use a sound meter for work on loudness levels. Sound meters are readily available from electronics stores and cost about $40 to $50 for basic models.

Summary

It might seem as if a chapter on phonation would be at the heart of a book on voice disorders. However, phonation itself is just one aspect of what needs to be addressed when a child has a voice disorder. The techniques discussed in this chapter help you address several specific problems with phonation.

Loudness Level Pictures

Choose either the library/classroom/playground or the mouse/cat/tiger pictures to represent loudness levels.

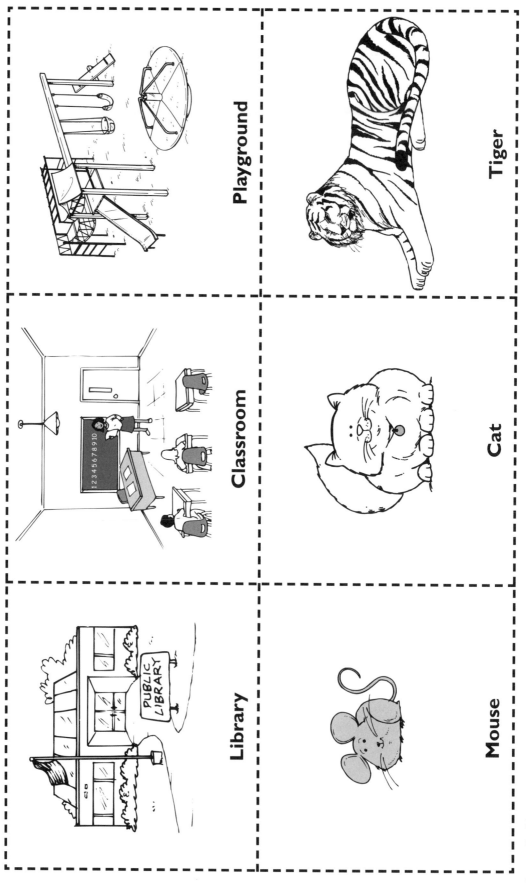

Library

Classroom

Playground

Mouse

Cat

Tiger

Appendix 8A
The Source for Children's Voice Disorders

The Loudness Match Game

Look at the small situation pictures. Match each small picture to the appropriate loudness level picture from Appendix 8A, page 126. Demonstrate the loudness level and tell why it is appropriate to use in that situation.

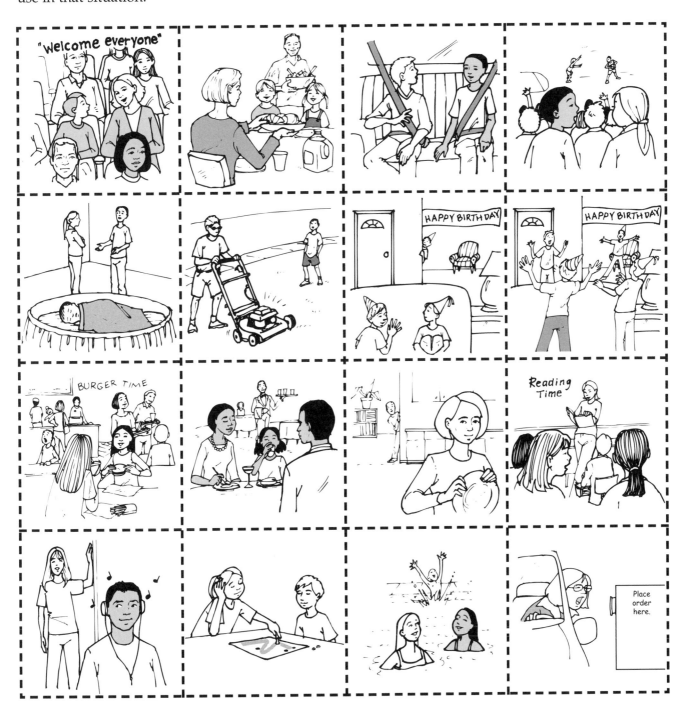

Record Form for Volume

Keep this form with you during the day. Write down each situation in which you talked. Then mark which loudness level you used in each situation. Bring this form back to your next therapy session and we'll talk about your choices.

Situation	Quiet	Medium	Loud

Pitch Picture Pairs

Use these pictures to talk about high and low pitch.

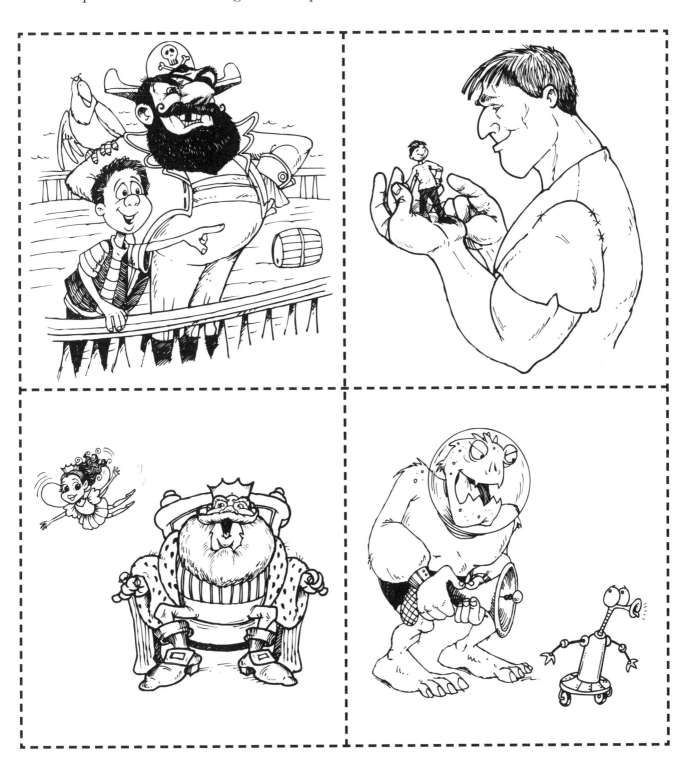

High and Low Pitch Characters

Use these pictures in pitch discrimination activities.

High Hank	High Hannah
Low Lou	**Low Louetta**

Vowel Words, Phrases, and Sentences

Say these words, phrases, and sentences using your target pitch.

One Syllable	Two Syllables	Three Syllables	Four Syllables
it	apple	animal	any day now
up	open	another	open it up
an	into	artistic	extra-special
in	other	example	easy does it
is	any	Alaska	information
on	about	announcing	experiment
as	away	area	experience
at	over	inside out	Indiana
if	after	estimate	inside the house
of	only	afternoon	unorganized
or	also	understand	Eat more apples.
all	again	exercise	identity
and	around	inspector	over and out
are	even	instrument	accelerate
one	under	already	Answer the phone.
use	always	exactly	Order more food.
us	along	addition	ecosystem
off	almost	Africa	under the bed
end	enough	indicate	Alabama
our	across	exciting	Oklahoma
old	order	industry	exercise here
air	easy	elevate	early to school
ask	early	umbrella	elevator
add	inside	elephant	application
eat	ocean	accident	Arizona
eye	ago	occupy	immediate
am	able	uniform	up and away
inch	island	electric	America
ice	explain	activate	identify
arm	object	emotion	Ask me for help.
act	include	important	up in the sky
ear	either	uppercase	already done
else	appear	objection	education
ate	outside	usual	enough playing
itch	ankle	engineer	unusual
age	earthquake	Idaho	illuminate
oak	empty	amigo	occupation
ace	occur	anyone	energetic
ink	absent	excellent	escalator
urge	untie	Ohio	Open the door.

Vowel Sentences

Say these sentences using your target pitch.

1. I like to go swimming in the lake.
2. All junk food is bad for growing children.
3. Am I going to be able to go fishing?
4. Anyone who wants to join the club can.
5. Are apples better than oranges?
6. Almost every girl wore pink to school on Friday.
7. Is Monday the first day of spring?
8. On the way to school, I studied my spelling words.
9. Every park in our town has fun playgrounds.
10. In the box was a fluffy bunny rabbit.
11. Up on the hill, there is a house.
12. A zebra can run very fast.
13. I left yesterday for space camp.
14. I am the farmer's son.
15. All of my friends are going to be there.
16. All is quiet tonight in the small village.
17. All of the boats sank during the hurricane.
18. Any child can learn to read.
19. "Am I pretty?" asked Grace.
20. Once you've told me, I won't forget.
21. Our teacher looked on as we worked.
22. Every seat in the theater was taken.
23. Every person turned toward the door.
24. Every once in a while, we get snow.
25. In Kentucky, basketball is very popular.
26. Amanda ate apples and bananas with her lunch.
27. Original copies of the book were stolen.
28. I like to take a nap in the afternoon.
29. Eight boats sailed across the sea.
30. Ocean waves pushed Abigail into the sandcastle.
31. Everyone needs an umbrella when it rains.
32. Elephants are bigger than zebras.
33. I have a friend who lives across the ocean.
34. Ask your teacher for help with your homework.
35. It is important to brush your teeth daily.

Onset Pairs

Use these pictures to contrast easy onset, hard attack, and breathy onset.

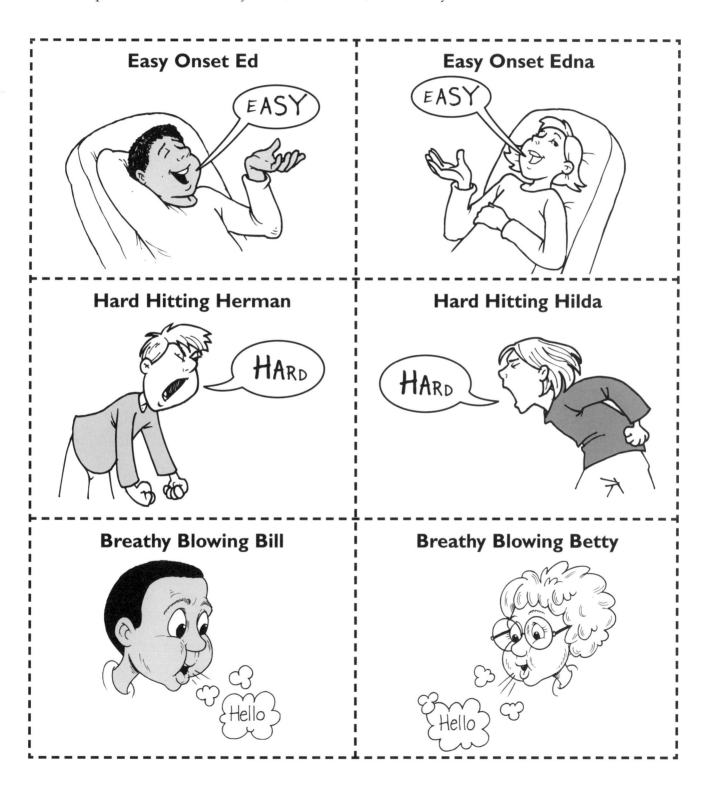

"H" Words

Say these words using an easy onset.

he	happy
head	hear
his	heart
horse	hill
have	hole
hold	history
had	human
how	hunt
heard	hit
her	hat
however	huge
him	habit
hundred	hair
has	hall
half	ham
house	hang
help	hello
hot	hero
home	hide
heat	hobby
hand	honey
heavy	hook
high	hope
held	hug
hard	hurry

Say these words using an easy onset.

arm	harm
and	hand
art	heart
am	ham
eat	heat
eel	heel
I've	hive
air	hair
all	hall
alter	halter
Andy	handy
arbor	harbor
as	has
ash	hash
at	hat
ate	hate
ugh	hug
edge	hedge
ear	hear
oaks	hoax
elm	helm
ill	hill
oh	hoe
is	his
it	hit
old	hold
owl	howl

Easy Onset Words and Sentences

Stop Consonants

Use easy onset on the vowel following the consonant.

Words	Sentences
pebbles	Pebbles hurt when they're in your shoe.
bananas	Bananas are a yellow fruit.
tomorrow	Tomorrow we will go on a trip.
dinosaurs	Dinosaurs like to eat leaves.
kingdoms	Kingdoms are full of fairies.
golf	Golf is a sport a lot of people like to play.
primary	Primary colors are bright colors.
birthday	Birthday parties are fun.
Tuesday	Tuesday is the best day of the week.
doctors	Doctors help sick people get well.

Voiceless Continuants

Use easy onset on the vowel following the consonant.

Words	Sentences
sunshine	Sunshine warms your face.
cheese	Cheese and crackers are a good snack.
shiny	Shiny pennies are fun to collect.
thanks	Thanks for helping me with my homework.
school	School starts in the fall.
children	Children love to play kickball.
shoes	Shoes are an important part of looking good.
fountain	Fountain water feels cool in the summer.
hardly	Hardly any fifth graders came to the play.
February	February is the month with Valentine's Day.

Voiced Continuants

Extend the consonant sound of the first word in each sentence.

Words	Sentences
many	Many of the students were late for class.
jumping	Jumping onto the trampoline is a lot of fun.
vines	Vines are growing on the side of the house.
zebras	Zebras are fast-running animals.
there	There are too many books on the shelf.
water	Water is the best thing to drink.
never	Never eat too much candy in one day.
lemonade	Lemonade tastes sour.
rabbits	Rabbits can hop fast.
jungles	Jungles are habitats for a lot of wild animals.

Appendix 8K
The Source for Children's Voice Disorders

9 | Oral-Nasal Resonance and Tone Focus

This chapter deals with two different concepts and descriptions of resonance. Each is included for different reasons. Each requires different approaches to therapy.

1. Hypernasality
2. Tone Focus

1. Hypernasality

When the term *resonance* is used in a narrow way to describe hypernasality, then resonance might be considered an articulation disorder rather than a voice disorder because it is caused by faulty movement and closure of an articulator, the soft palate. Why, then, does a book on voice disorders address hypernasality?

This book addresses hypernasality briefly because hypernasality can be associated with voice disorders, particularly in certain populations. For example, children with velopharyngeal insufficiency who have hypernasality may develop a voice disorder because they use excess muscle tension when phonating in an effort to compensate for air escaping through the nose. Most hypernasality is caused by a structural problem that likely needs surgical intervention. Perhaps the child has already received surgical intervention with some remaining hypernasality that may respond to therapy.

Another example of the relationship between voice and hypernasality might be seen in a child who has a hyperfunctional voice disorder with tension in oropharyngeal musculature. This child might use very little mouth movement during speech and thus be perceived as somewhat hypernasal. This would be a purely functional cause of hypernasality.

This book does not deal in depth with hypernasality due to structural, organic causes (e.g., cleft palate). The discussion of hypernasality in this book is focused on children who have a mild-moderate perceived hypernasality (whether the result of a structural or functional reason) that should respond to therapeutic approaches. If the cause is organic, such as repaired cleft, and all surgical interventions have been performed, then the residual hypernasality might be addressed as a functional problem to see if the child can make other changes to reduce the perception of hypernasality. A short-term goal and treatment objectives for addressing this hypernasality are listed in the box on the next page.

2. Tone Focus

Where does the voice sound like it comes from?

The more pertinent description of resonance, however, relates to the overall focus of the child's speech and voice. There is a significant interaction between phonation and resonance. The voice (phonation produced at the level of the larynx) is altered by how it resonates throughout all of the supralaryngeal structures. Not only does an acceptable voice require a balance between perceived oral and nasal resonance as described above, it also requires that the voice be "placed" accurately in the oral cavity. One problem that can be observed with resonance of phonation within the oral cavity is that caused by carrying the tongue too far forward or too far back in the oral cavity. If the tongue is held in a high, forward position, the resonance is often described as a thin or baby-sounding voice. Conversely, a tongue carried in the back of the mouth is described as cul-de-sac resonance. This may be observed in children who are deaf or may be part of a hyperfunctional voice disorder. The term *tone focus* is often used to describe where the resonance is occurring in the oral-pharyngeal region.

Another frequent problem with tone focus is the child who sounds as if his voice is coming directly out of his throat. That is, the child is not correctly focusing the tone of his voice in the area of the nose and cheek. This appropriate area of focus was called "placing the voice" by Boone et al. (2005). It may also be called "speaking from the mask area" (visualize an oxygen mask). A voice that instead is focused in the throat sounds gravelly and low-pitched. A focus in the throat may be associated with hyperfunction/muscle tension dysphonia. This type of misplaced focus is also a resonance issue.

A short-term goal and treatment objectives for working on appropriate resonance in oral cavity and in the mask area are listed on the next page.

Short-term Goal

Child will eliminate misuse of resonance and instead will focus the phonation/tone appropriately within the mouth and nose area (MU-TFR)

Treatment Objectives

1. Child will discriminate between thin (forward focus), muffled (cul-de-sac) resonance and appropriately balanced oral resonance when modeled by SLP. (MU-TFR-1)

2. Child will discriminate between thin (forward focus), muffled (cul-de-sac) resonance and appropriately balanced oral resonance in audiotape/live samples of own speech. (MU-TFR-2)

3. Child will utilize resonance that is balanced between the front and back of the mouth on/in: (MU-TFR-3)

   a. vowels (MU-TFR-3a)

   b. words (MU-TFR-3b)

   c. phrases and sentences (MU-TFR-3c)

   d. conversation (MU-TFR-3d)

4. Child will discriminate between phonation/tone focused in the throat and that focused in the mouth and nose area when modeled by SLP. (MU-TFR-4)

5. Child will discriminate between phonation/tone focused in the throat and that focused in the mouth and nose area in audiotape/live samples of own speech. (MU-TFR-5)

6. Child will utilize resonance that is appropriately focused in the mouth and nose area on/in: (MU-TFR-6)

   a. vowels (MU-TFR-6a)

   b. words (MU-TFR-6b)

   c. phrases and sentences (MU-TFR-6c)

   d. conversation (MU-TFR-6d)

Hypernasality related to cleft palate

The most common organic cause of hypernasality is cleft palate. Treating organic resonance problems such as those related to clefts is typically approached through surgery, orthodontics, and prosthodontics. However, sometimes after the surgery and any orthodontic work or placement of a prosthesis, the child still is perceived as somewhat hypernasal. Some of the techniques described below might be worth trying in a short trial of therapy to determine if this perceived hypernasality can be reduced.

Hypernasality following removal of tonsils and adenoids

Sometimes following a tonsillectomy and adenoidectomy, a child sounds hypernasal. This may be because a new structural problem has been created as a result of the surgery. There may be two reasons for this structural change.

1. The child's soft palate is too short to contact the pharyngeal walls in the absence of adenoidal tissue. Therapy is not likely to help this child.

2. The child's palate may be of adequate length to contact the posterior pharyngeal wall, but he needs to learn to move the soft palate more to reach the pharyngeal walls. This is a functional resonance problem, and therapy would be indicated.

Functional hypernasality

Sometimes there may be no apparent organic reason for a child to sound hypernasal. Certain regional dialects within the United States contain more hypernasality than others. If you think a child sounds hypernasal and have ruled out that any organic problem might be causing the perception, then you might try treating this child's hypernasality as a functional problem. Hypernasality is a difficult problem to fix, and if the child and the child's parents don't "hear" it as a problem, the prognosis for change is not good.

Discrimination of Hypernasal Resonance

MU-ONR Treatment Objective 1	Child will discriminate oral vs. hypernasal resonance as modeled by SLP.

MU-ONR Treatment Objective 2	Child will discriminate between oral and nasal resonance in audiotape/live samples of own speech.

The first thing the child has to do is discriminate what you mean by hypernasal resonance vs. appropriate resonance. Provide exaggerated models of hypernasal speech, hyponasal speech, and speech with a balanced resonance. This is difficult for some clinicians to do, so you should practice before trying this in front of the child. To produce hypernasal sounding speech, let your soft palate hang relaxed so that all the sound goes "into your nose." You can utilize assimilation to help you do this by using a sentence containing a lot of nasal phonemes as you try to mimic hypernasality. The high vowels /i/ and /u/ will make you sound more nasal (e.g., "Many mean men meet at Moon's on Monday.").

To produce hyponasal speech, pretend that you have a cold. Using a sentence with no nasal phonemes will help with this task. Do this by holding the soft palate in an elevated position so that no sound can go into the nasal cavity. A sentence with no nasal phonemes and no high vowels can help you produce hyponasal speech (e.g., "Bob the dog hopped on the porch."). You can also pinch your nostrils shut to produce an approximation of hyponasal speech.

You can play an audiotape sample of the child's hypernasal speech compared to some audiotape samples of same age and gender peers who have appropriate resonance so that the child can hear the difference. If the child's hypernasality is more easily perceived in assimilative contexts, the sentences loaded with nasal phonemes in Appendix 9B, pages 148-149, may come in handy. (Note: This is the same appendix used in the "I've got a cold" technique on page 141.)

Techniques to reduce hypernasality

MU-ONR Treatment Objective 3	Child will reduce perceived hypernasality on/in: a. vowels b. words c. phrases and sentences d. conversation

Any or all of the strategies described below may be helpful to a particular child in reducing the perception of hypernasality. The treatment objectives are written in a hierarchy, starting with production of something easy (e.g., vowel sounds) and progressing toward using the new pattern of resonance in conversational speech. Appendix 9A, page 147, lists each of these approaches.

1. I've got a cold

Stemple et al. (2000) point out that sometimes you should try the most obvious approach first. They suggest you talk with the child about modeling a voice that sounds as if you have a cold and seeing if the child can utilize this technique. The sentences in Appendix 9B, pages 148-149, may be helpful for this activity. The first set of sentences has no nasal phonemes. These may be the easiest for the child to use at first. The second set has many nasal phonemes. The child may need to pinch his nose at first to be able to produce them without nasality. The third set of sentences contains a balance of nasal and non-nasal phonemes.

2. Reducing rate

Some children talk so fast that they literally don't give their articulators time to move. Slowing the child's rate may help the child with the next strategy (over-articulating). One way to practice reducing rate is to have the child tap the table or his leg as he says each word. This can be done with sentences, reading material, or even during conversation.

3. Over-articulating

If the child speaks with too little mouth movement, the voice may resonate more in the nasal cavity because the child is not opening the oral cavity (Wilson 1979). Demonstrate to the child how you can change your resonance simply by over articulating and moving your mouth as compared to keeping your jaw and teeth tightly closed what you speak. Sit in front of the mirror so the child can watch your mouth and his mouth at the same time. Appendix 9C, pages 150-151, contains words and sentences with open vowels. These may be helpful to use to encourage the child to begin to use more mouth movement.

4. Changing the pitch

Boone et al. (2005) indicate that some children with hypernasality speak with a pitch that is too high. Lowering the pitch may change the perception of hypernasality. See Chapter 8, pages 121-122, for techniques to alter pitch.

Utilizing instrumentation as biofeedback

The child may benefit from using instrumentation so he can see how his productions change. Kay Elemetrics makes a *Nasometer* that is useful for this purpose.

Tone Focus in the Mouth

If the child is holding his tongue too far forward or back within the oral cavity, resonance can be affected.

Discrimination of tongue carriage effect on tone focus

MU-TFR Treatment Objective 1	Child will discriminate between thin (forward focus), muffled (cul-de-sac) resonance and appropriately balanced oral resonance when modeled by SLP.
MU-TFR Treatment Objective 2	Child will discriminate between thin (forward focus), muffled (cul-de-sac) resonance and appropriately balanced oral resonance in audiotape/live samples of own speech.

The child must be able to discriminate the impact that carriage of the tongue too far forward or too far back in the mouth has on the overall tone focus or resonance of the voice. You may need to model these two tongue carriage positions for the child so he can hear the difference. The thin-sounding voice produced by tongue carriage too far forward in the mouth can be simulated by reducing mouth opening and keeping the tongue tip up and forward near the alveolar ridge. To simulate the production of a cul-de-sac resonance, pull the tongue farther back into the oral cavity and keep it there as phonemes are produced.

Techniques to achieve accurate placement of the tongue in the oral cavity

MU-TFR Treatment Objective 3	Child will utilize resonance that is balanced between the front and back of the mouth on/in: a. vowels b. words c. phrases and sentences d. conversation

If the child is carrying the tongue too far forward in the mouth, resulting in a thin quality to the vocal resonance, have the child practice sentences that have back vowels and back-of-the-mouth phonemes to encourage more accurate tongue placement. Appendix 9D, page 152, contains some phrases and sentences to practice.

If, instead, the child is producing a cul-de-sac resonance with the tongue pulled too far back in the oral cavity, production of sentences with alveolar consonants and even bilabials paired with front vowels may help the child produce better resonance. Appendix 9E, page 153, has some stimuli for this practice. The child may have some success with over-articulation and increased movement of the mouth. Sentences beginning with open vowels may encourage this over-articulation. (See Appendix 9C, pages 150-151.)

Tone Focus in the Mask

The lesson that many children need to learn about tone focus is how to get the voice out of the throat and up into the head. Teaching the child how to focus the resonance of the voice in the mask area is a technique often used for children with hyperfunctional voice disorders and for children who have pitch problems.

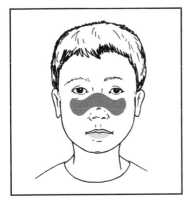

As Stemple et al. (2000) explain, when the vocal tract is relaxed and open with no obstructions above the level of the glottis, the tone can resonate freely. This may be described as having a "forward focus" or placement of the tone. When the child is exhibiting tension at any point in the vocal tract, there will be a change in the resonance of the tone and the vocal quality. This change in where the tone is placed may also create a voice that fatigues easily.

Discriminating focus in the mask area

MU-TFR Treatment Objective 4	Child will discriminate between phonation/tone focused in the throat and that focused in the mouth and nose area when modeled by SLP.
MU-TFR Treatment Objective 5	Child will discriminate between phonation/tone focused in the throat and that focused in the mouth and nose area in audiotape/live samples of own speech.

To help the child discriminate between the voice that has the tone focused appropriately in the area of the nose in the mouth, called the *mask area*, to a voice that is focused in the throat, you will need to use good examples and visualization techniques. Model some phrases for the child using one of these areas of focus and see if the child can tell you whether you are using your mask voice or your throat voice. If this is difficult for the child, start by producing the sound "m" or a word like *me* repetitively, and have the child feel the vibrations across the bridge of your nose. Contrast this with production of the same sound or word produced in a more guttural, low-pitched way to demonstrate the throat voice.

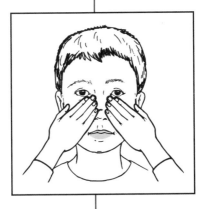

When the child seems reliable in discriminating these two types of productions when you model them, see if you can provide examples within the child's own speech of each of these types of focus. The child may not currently be using any speech that is appropriately focused in the nose and mouth area, but will surely provide you with examples of a throat voice. Listen carefully at the end of each of the child's utterances, as it is common for children to drop their pitch and their focus as they run out of air toward the end of the sentence. To help the child contrast this with appropriate tone focus, have the child place his fingers near the bridge of his nose while he hums so that he can feel the vibrations.

Other techniques that may help the child become more aware of focusing sound on the lips as well as in the nasal cavity have been described. Stemple et al. (2000) uses lip trills and tongue trills. A lip trill is also known as a *raspberry*, or a *motorcycle noise* (but make sure the child is not adding phonation to the sound made by the lips). A tongue trill is made by trilling the tongue against the alveolar ridge rapidly. Wrap wax paper around a comb and hold this against the lips while the child produces the lip trill or an "m" sound.

Changing focus to the mask area

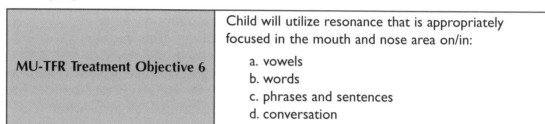

MU-TFR Treatment Objective 6	Child will utilize resonance that is appropriately focused in the mouth and nose area on/in: a. vowels b. words c. phrases and sentences d. conversation

Many authors have written about the importance of changing the tone focus to an area in the front of the face (Lessac 1973, Stemple et al. 2000, Verdolini 1998; Boone et al. 2005, Rammage et al. 2001, Andrews and Summers 2002). This work on tone focus has been called *placing the voice, resonance enhancement, resonance voice therapy, nasalized phrase production,* and *chanting,* among other descriptions. A review of these multiple descriptions yields the following suggestions for a step-by-step approach to help the child change the focus of the resonance from the throat to the face. Appendix 9F, page 154, lists the steps so you can keep track of how the child is doing.

1. Nasal phonemes

With the child's fingers on the bridge of his nose, ask him to produce nasal phonemes with you. Encourage the child to exaggerate the vibrations in the nose as he produces these sounds. Monitor to make sure the child is not also using a guttural, forced production of these phonemes. If that is the case, ask the child to produce the nasal phonemes at a slightly higher pitch to encourage the change in tone focus. You can also have the child produce an "h" and "m" together ("hmmm") or "h" and "n" together ("hnnn") to eliminate the hard glottal attack on the "m." Use any verbal descriptions or visual imagery techniques to help the child understand what you mean by changing where the voice is placed.

2. Vowel sounds

You may want to begin by using the high front vowel /i/ that should encourage placement in the front of the mouth. Have the child imitate the /i/ in a very nasalized way. Model the difference in the nasal vs. non-nasal /i/. During all of these vocalizations, be sure to encourage the child not to force the sound but to produce it lightly and easily upon exhalation.

3. Syllables for chanting

Combine one of the nasal phonemes with this high front vowel /i/ for a repetitious chant "mee-mee-mee-mee-mee," keeping the sound focused in the nasal cavity. If the child has difficulty, remind him that he is simply continuing to make the /i/ and just opening and closing his lips. You can try other chants such as "nee-nee-nee-nee-nee" and "meany-meany-meany-meany." You can also use other vowels in the syllable with the nasal phoneme. These chants are typically done on one note. Tell the child that you want these to sound like they are staying on one note. That is, you do not want these produced in the talking voice but in a chanting, humming voice.

4. Varying parameters of chanting

Before making the transition to using this new tone focus for words, help the child gain some control by practicing changing different parameters (i.e., pitch, rate, loudness) (Stemple 2000). You may need to practice each of these parameters to make sure the child understands what you mean by *slower*, *faster*, *softer*, *louder*, *higher*, and *lower*. If the child can make all changes except the latter two (changes in pitch), then just focus on the changes he can easily make. Appendix 9G, page 155, provides visual cues to help the child as he practices.

At first, just change one of the parameters. For example, have the child chant the phrase "meany-meany-meany-meany" and then change the rate so he's going faster. If he can manage this and still maintain the good tone focus, you might ask him to go faster and a little louder or faster and a little softer. Depending on the age of the child, you may only want to ask for one parameter to be changed. Use the pictures in Appendix 9G to cue the child about the change you want made.

5. Words beginning with nasal phonemes

When the child has mastered chanting with some changes in at least several parameters, have the child produce words that begin with the nasal phonemes. Have the child prolong the nasal phoneme for a second or two so that he can hear that he has the sound focused appropriately in the mask area. Then the child can open his mouth to produce the rest of the word. The words should be produced on one note so the child can concentrate on where the tone is focused and not the inflectional pattern (that's the next step!). For example, the word *made* would sound like "mmmmmade." Words beginning with nasal phonemes are listed in Appendix 9H, page 156.

6. Phrases beginning with nasal phonemes

At first, the child should produce these phrases on a single note, just like he was doing with the words. This allows him to continue to concentrate on where the tone is focused and not worry about the inflectional pattern. Also, the child may have a tendency to drop the focus into the throat near the end of the utterance. Therefore he needs more practice on keeping the entire phrase focused in the mask area. The child may need to continue to extend the nasal phoneme for a second or two before producing the rest of the phrase.

When the child has achieved some mastery at this level, you can ask him to shift into a "sing-song" pattern. That means that the child will:

- hold the nasal phoneme for second or two
- finish that word on the same note
- move to a sing-song inflectional pattern to finish the phrase

The challenge may occur as you transition to having the child produce the phrases with normal intonation. You can use negative practice to help the child with this step.

Have the child produce a phrase in the sing-song inflectional pattern with good tone focus in the mask area. Contrast with a phrase produced in a guttural fashion with focus in the throat. Appendix 9H (page 156) lists phrases and sentences for practice.

7. Other phrases and sentences

Presenting stimuli that do not begin with the nasal phoneme may make it a little more difficult for the child to achieve the appropriate tone focus. If the child has difficulty, revert to the sing-song pattern or even to having the child produce the entire phrase on one note to help him regain the tone focus.

8. Conversation

Engage the child in conversation and help him learn how to monitor where his resonance is focused. If you find the child is slipping, return to an earlier step to help the child regain focus.

Summary

Teaching the child to change the placement of the tongue in the oral cavity for better resonance, or to change the focus of the resonance from the throat to the mask area of the face, is challenging. Reducing the perception of hypernasality may be the trickiest of all. Lots of modeling, imagery, and practice will be needed. Helping the child transfer the use of the new resonance pattern to situations outside the therapy setting is an important last step to generalization of the new pattern. All of this work pays off when the child sounds better and his vocal mechanism is healthier.

Oral and Nasal Resonance Balance

Name _____

▷ I'm practicing to make my speech resonance sound balanced.

_____ Talking through my nose

_____ Talking from my mouth

▷ I'm using these techniques.

_____ Pretending I have a cold

_____ Slowing down

_____ Moving my mouth when I speak

_____ Using my lower voice

Please help me remember to use them!

Sentences With/Without Nasal Phonemes

Sentences without *m*, *n*, or *ng* words

1. All of the boys brought bread to the party.
2. Every day our teacher tells us what to do.
3. Each girl waited for her father to arrive.
4. I like to eat carrots for breakfast.
5. Bobbie will be six years old April 1st.
6. He got Allie a puppy for her birthday.
7. Geri studied social studies for two hours.
8. Chico's cat was sick after it had its shots.
9. Takisha brought chocolate cake for dessert.
10. Pedro forgot to stop at the store.
11. Todd was very sleepy after basketball practice.
12. Paula would choose baseball over basketball.
13. We had eight eggs for breakfast.
14. Pizza is the best food for supper.
15. Jared took a big juicy bite of the apple.
16. Carla put away the boxes she liked.
17. I wear white socks with red shoes.
18. Rico's backpack was very heavy.
19. A rabbit hopped swiftly toward the bush.
20. Jake likes to eat jelly with his biscuits.
21. Teachers have to grade a lot of papers.
22. For the field trip, the class traveled to the city zoo.
23. Australia is a good place to see whales.
24. The girl huffed as she pedaled up the hill.
25. Grover is the fluffy cat without a tail.

Sentences with *m*, *n*, or *ng* words

1. I never know how Maddie balances so many things.
2. My knees knock now and then.
3. My friend Madison often moans and groans on Mondays.
4. I think my mom mailed me a box in November.
5. Karen didn't return Marty's math book on time.
6. Mr. Norman ran out of nails when he built his new fence.
7. Mario beamed as he admired his new haircut.
8. Monkeys must drink a lot of milk to be so strong.
9. Nina and Maya are not friends any more.
10. Matty might make muffins for his morning meal.
11. My mother saw a moose in the mountains.
12. Mike went shopping at the market this morning.
13. Nona made nine more necklaces.

14. To make moist cake, mix the milk with melted butter.
15. You will need nine men and women to make one snowman.
16. Ramon doesn't like living near the mean neighbor.
17. Most monsters make noise at night.
18. My animals are never napping at noon.
19. Never mail macaroni noodles to Frank in Mexico.
20. Thomas thinks that summer is better than winter.
21. It took many minutes for Jamal to find the umbrella.
22. One thing that no one missed was math homework.
23. Emma enjoyed making Malika a meal.
24. Can Amanda and Jamie come over on Monday evening?
25. Something is making an annoying noise in the basement.

Balanced sentences (2-4 words have *m*, *n*, or *ng*)

1. Did you ever want to see a lion or a snake?
2. How many students got to go to the park?
3. Whenever my sister wakes up in the night, she cries.
4. Do you want to open a savings account?
5. Most people want a fancy cake for a wedding.
6. Manatees are easy-going animals.
7. Mamiko likes to play with pretend make-up.
8. I finally got all of my math problems right.
9. My best friend moved away yesterday morning.
10. It is boring to wait a long time.
11. I don't understand my math teacher.
12. I like to enjoy a movie while eating popcorn.
13. I like to add mustard to my sandwiches.
14. During summer, I will turn eleven years old.
15. Karen thought her puppy was her most important present.
16. Tonya ran over a nail in the road so she got a flat tire.
17. Makalo and her dad love baseball very much.
18. Mom forgot to stop at the store to buy milk and muffins.
19. One thing many children do is make their beds.
20. You go to a hardware store to buy nails.
21. Mario looked at the comic book and smiled.
22. Check the newspaper for times of new movies.
23. Hank found the missing sock in his drawer.
24. Mrs. Smith's favorite animals at the zoo were the monkeys.
25. Reading a magazine can be very relaxing.

Words and Sentences with Open Vowels

Words

short o

honest
honor
honor roll
honorable
object
obligation
oblong
observation
obsolete
obstacle
obvious
occupant
occupy

octagon
October
octopus
odd
oddity
odyssey
off
offense
offer
offering
offhand
office
offline

offset
often
olive
Oliver
omelet
on
ongoing
online
onto
onyx
opera
opportunity

opposite
opposition
optical
optimistic
option
ostrich
otter
ottoman
ox
oxidize
oxygen
Oz

au/aw

auburn
auction
audible
audience
audio
audiology
audiometer
audit
audition

auditor
auditory
Audubon
augment
August
Aussie
austere
Austin
Australia

Austria
authentic
author
authority
authorize
autism
autistic
autobiography
automatic

automobile
autopsy
autumn
auxiliary
awe
awesome
awful
awkward
awning

uh

await
awake
awaken
award
aware
away
awhile
awoke
udder
ugly
ultimate
ultra
umbrella

umpire
unable
unarmed
unaware
unbelievable
unbend
unbind
unbroken
unbutton
uncap
uncertain
uncle
uncomfortable

uncut
under
underachieve
undercover
undercut
underfoot
underhand
underneath
underpass
undersea
undershirt
understand

understanding
underwater
underwrite
undo
undress
uneasy
up
upbeat
upper
upstream
usher
utter

Sentences

1. October is an awesome month.
2. Always remember that opposites attract.
3. Umbrellas are often useful.
4. Understudies understand how to play the part.
5. Ugly ducklings don't live under the sea.
6. Automobiles parked under awnings stay cool in the summer.
7. An octopus would never be friends with an ox.
8. I awake at eight to unbutton my shirt.
9. Uncomfortable shoes are often worn in Australia.
10. Office supplies include odds and ends.
11. An obstacle doesn't automatically mean you have to stop.
12. Almost all audiences clap at the end of *Sleeping Beauty*.
13. Upper shelves are often hard for Olivia to reach.
14. Austin was unaware that he was on the Honor Roll.
15. Uncle Luis is an umpire for Oliver's baseball team.
16. Omelets are the ultimate breakfast meal.
17. Unbroken objects were found upstream.
18. Authors like to go away to deserted islands.
19. Olives are good on cheese pizza.
20. Ostriches and otters are often unbelievable animals.
21. Honesty is always the best approach.
22. August and autumn are almost here.
23. Offer the award to the usher.
24. Observing the operation made me uneasy.
25. Austin was unable to throw underhand.
26. An octagon is not an oblong shape.
27. Undercover agents have to be optimistic.
28. Undershirts obviously keep babies warm.
29. Ongoing projects were put underneath the table.
30. I awoke to the audible sound of birds.
31. Offer to sit on the ottoman.
32. Audiotapes were being auctioned for two dollars.
33. Underachievers were in awe when the boat sank.
34. Awkward moments often occur in an opera.
35. Aware of the danger, I chose not to climb onto the ladder.

Phrases and Sentences with Back Vowels and Back Consonants

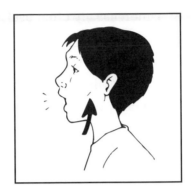

1. Can you carry the card for Carlos?
2. Hug your granny and give her a kiss.
3. The huge hog put his snout in the mud.
4. Hang your cool coat on the hook in the nook.
5. Sailing in tugboats is cool while drinking cups of cola.
6. How awful was the waffle that Gaspar cooked?
7. Kirk owes me money for cleaning the outside awning.
8. Kayla hugged the kid dressed as a king.
9. Good girls cook grits for their great grandmas at breakfast.
10. Bang the gong that hangs above the ring.
11. Harold has hair on his head.
12. My coat was left in the back of the canoe.
13. Ken is in the mood to eat lots of good food.
14. I took a good look at that huge book.
15. August is an awful time for an opera or audition.
16. Carlita eats canned food while camping.
17. I was glad to get the graduation gift.
18. Harriet the hog hates hamburgers.
19. I was shook up after Makalo kicked the desk.
20. Don't groan while shopping for coats.
21. The author awoke at the auction.
22. Could the girls carry the huge hangers?
23. Olive was unable to achieve the goal.
24. Oliver is always honest and optimistic.
25. Carrie's back hurt from sitting on the awful ottoman.
26. The cardboard carton broke when Kyle kicked it.
27. Carl scored a goal during the soccer game.
28. Harry owns two collie dogs.
29. Lagoons are full of frogs and bugs.
30. Greg likes to eat grapes for breakfast.
31. The swimming pool was cold because of all the rain.
32. I like to look through books about gorillas.
33. Hank goes camping every holiday.
34. Carmen hates to eat hamburgers.
35. Chris sang in the holiday concert.

Phrases and Sentences with Front Vowels and Front Consonants

1. Tiny Tim danced on top of the tiny table.
2. Don't hit it; just tap the top of Nellie's boot.
3. Talid and Latoya didn't want to tell Tom.
4. Dancing doesn't make Laura seem dignified.
5. Lilly likes learning new languages.
6. Never nag about napping at noon.
7. Daniel puts peanut butter on pickles.
8. Making muffins with mom is fun.
9. Big boys play baseball with big bats.

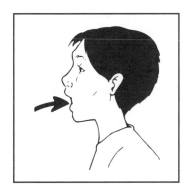

10. Four frogs had fun playing in the fog.
11. On vacation, Victor and his family looked for a place with vacant rooms.
12. Never be late for an important date.
13. My best tie is loaded with cat hair.
14. Too many tigers escaped from the zoo.
15. Do you like decorating dance halls?
16. The movie theater had lots of long lines to buy tickets.
17. Nina knocked at the door nine times.
18. Put plenty of powder on the paper.
19. Mothers make mornings more remarkable.
20. Taking a bath brings up bad behavior.
21. Foolish friends fight over food.
22. The villain liked to eat vanilla ice cream.
23. Thomas had to sit in the corner after having a tantrum.
24. Tina met Ed at a bread eating contest.
25. Lavon was late for the date.
26. My seat at the swim meet was wet.
27. Tim's pet ate all of his plants.
28. Ted did not take pictures of Mr. Leet.
29. Apple pie is a good summer dessert.
30. Lucy won a bike on her birthday.
31. Dragons breathe fire when they are mad.
32. The students take a spelling test every Tuesday.
33. Tammy likes to dine at nine.
34. My dog licked Pete's lollipop.
35. Marcos made muffins with the twins.

Steps of Tone Focus

Name _____

I am learning how to project my voice from the mask area (my nose and mouth).

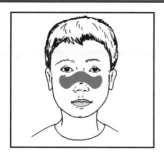

These are the steps I am practicing:

1. ☐ Humming nose sounds ("mmmm" "nnnn")

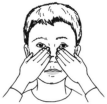

2. ☐ Making vowel sounds in my nose ("eeee")

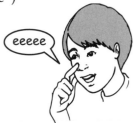

3. ☐ Chanting syllables with nose sounds
    mee-mee-mee
    nee-nee-nee-nee
    moe-moe-moe
    my-moe-my-moe-my-moe
    my knee, my knee, my knee
    me-oh-my, me-oh-my, me-oh-my
    meany, meany, meany
    May I, May I, May I

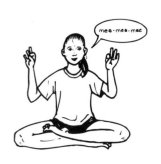

4. ☐ Chanting with change (fast, slow, high, low)

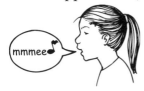

5. ☐ Words with nose sounds on one note (see list in Appendix 9B)

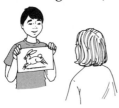

6. ☐ Phrases with nose sounds on one note (see list in Appendix 9B)

☐ Phrases with nose sounds sing-song (see list in Appendix 9B)

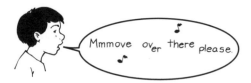

☐ Other phrases sing-song (see lists in Appendices 9B, 9D, and 9E)

7. ☐ Phrases regular (see lists in Appendices 9B, 9D, and 9E)

Changing the Parameters of Speech

These pictures can help the child understand how to change the parameters of phonation: fast vs. slow, high vs. low, and loud vs. soft.

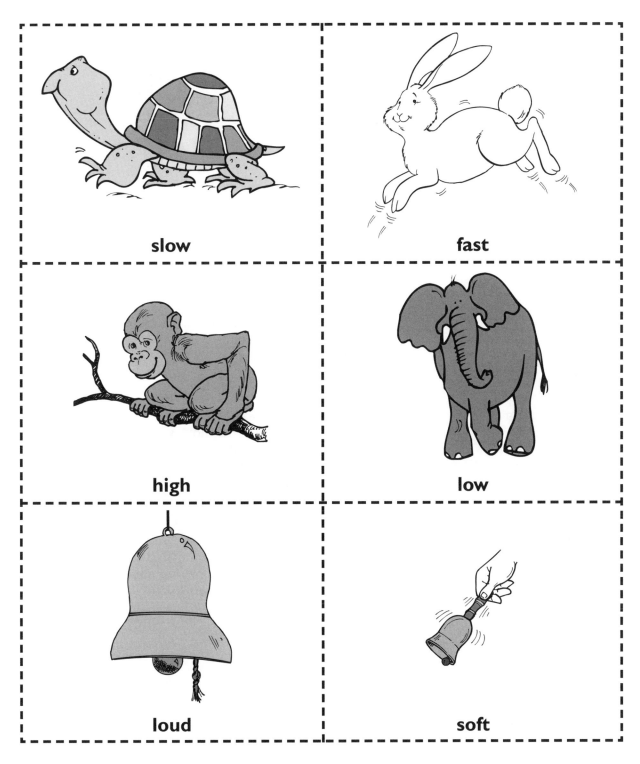

slow

fast

high

low

loud

soft

Words, Phrases, and Sentences Beginning with *"m"* or *"n"*

Words

man	mix	might	much
not	near	mouth	move
make	need	master	nickel
meal	meet	may	nothing
never	napkin	now	mother
monkey	milk	more	nation
news	nest	made	magic
next	night	number	money
mom	neck	new	neglect
nine	normal	necessary	magnet

Phrases and Sentences

Meet my mom.
Never nap at night.
Newt knows names.
Mix more milk.
need nine naps
never nest near
March for a mile.
need a new nose
Mark my mailbag.
Moths make a mess.
nine napkins for me
next news at nine
no new news
Make more movies.
notice nine notes
muddy men move
nuts in the nests
Nate or Nicholas
Monkeys make messes.
noon not nine

Mice might make money.
noodles on napkins
Nadia napped.
Nita made milk.
Mikey milked many cows.
Marcos munched muffins.
Mori marched to Minnesota.
Never knot a napkin.
Nothing needs to go next.
master mechanics
Meet me at the movies.
normal nights are near
Miranda likes melted muffins.
more milk for Malik
number one nickel
Mothers make muffins.
May I mow the lawn?
Nieces and nephews need to know.
Musicians know many notes.
Move over there please.

Paradoxical Vocal Fold Dysfunction (PVFD)

Paradoxical Vocal Fold Dysfunction (PVFD) is known by many other names, most commonly *Vocal Cord Dysfunction* (VCD) or *Paradoxical Vocal Fold Motion*. Other descriptors include emotional laryngeal wheezing, chronic acute laryngospasms, functional airway obstruction, factitious asthma, and episodic paryoxysmal laryngospasm. PVFD is not a voice disorder, though a small percentage of clients may present with related hoarseness. Why then is a chapter on PVFD included in a book on voice disorders in children? It seems a logical place to share such information since knowledge of the respiratory and phonatory anatomy and physiology is crucial to diagnosing and treating PVFD, and since SLPs play a crucial role in its treatment. SLPs can also educate others about this often misdiagnosed disorder.

What Is PVFD?

The normal position of the vocal folds during inspiration and expiration is in an open position during inspiration and only slightly less open position during expiration. The paradoxical motion of the vocal folds that occurs during PVFD is a tight adduction of the vocal folds during the inspiratory cycle. The vocal folds are in the shape of a Y with a small chink at the posterior edges.

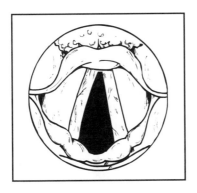 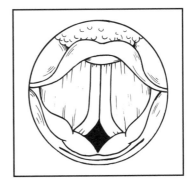

The paradoxical adduction can sometimes occur during the expiratory cycle as well. This adduction leads to obstruction of airflow with wheezing and sometimes stridor.

The etiology of PVFD is unknown, though it may be related to neurologic, psychologic, or structural disorders. A lot of patients with PVFD also have GERD (see page 56) and therefore GERD may be a possible etiologic factor, as may postnasal drip or sinusitis (Perkner et al. 1998, Powell et al. 2000).

There is no information on prevalence. It can begin at any age but seems to be most common between the ages of 10 and 40 (Kuppersmith et al. 1993). However, there are reports of it occurring in infants (Heatley & Swift 1996). In children, it occurs three times more in girls than boys (Newman et al. 1995). In an excellent tutorial presented in the *American Journal of Speech-Language Pathology*, Mathers-Schmidt (2001) suggests that this disorder should be viewed as "a complex, heterogeneous disorder in both its etiology and expression" (p. 112).

What are the symptoms?

Children with PVFD may present with the following symptoms:

- stridor or noisy breathing when breathing in
- wheezing
- difficulty swallowing
- shortness of breath
- hoarseness
- tightness in throat or upper chest
- sensation of choking

These symptoms typically occur episodically. In children, they are often associated with sports. They may occur related to anxiety (e.g., test taking) but this is more common in adolescents than younger children. It may be seen more frequently in high achievers (Brugman & Newman 1993). In adults, psychological factors and exposure to airway irritants may be etiologic.

Misdiagnosed as asthma

Because of the episodic nature of PVFD, the restricted airflow and respiratory sounds that accompany PVFD, it may be confused with asthma (Christopher et al. 1983). Many times the child will have a diagnosis of *asthma unresponsive to therapy*. This means that the child has been prescribed bronchodilators and steroids and has not benefited from their use. Sometimes children have had multiple trips to the emergency room and even hospitalizations when they have one of their attacks (Tan et al. 1997). The inability to breathe in can cause a child to feel as if she is going to die.

Children can also be thought to have exercise-induced asthma (EIA) when it is really exercise-induced PVFD. There are some differences in how these symptoms present. With PVFD, symptoms occur suddenly and within a few minutes of beginning the exercise. Symptoms usually subside fairly quickly when the child stops exercising (Landwehr et al. 1996). This is different from EIA where it usually takes the symptoms 5 to 10 minutes to develop after intense exercise and it takes much longer (15-30 minutes) for the symptoms to resolve (Storms 1999).

Related factors

As mentioned above, many patients who have PVFD also have GERD. The acid refluxed from the stomach may enter the upper airway and splash on the vocal folds, causing a protective closing action. One small study found that 19 of 22 children with PVFD had evidence of GERD (Powell et al. 2000). If the history indicates any possibility that the child might have GERD, it is crucial that it be managed in order to control the symptoms of PVFD. If the child complains that he wakes up unable to breathe in the middle of the night, it is usually GERD that is triggering the attacks.

Although PVFD is often misdiagnosed as asthma, these two disorders can co-occur (Caraon & O'Toole 1991, Warburton et al. 1996). If the child has both, teaching him techniques to open the adducted larynx before he reaches for his bronchodilator will help deliver more of the medication to the lungs where it is needed. If the child tries to breathe in the asthma medications while the vocal folds are tightly adducted, not much of the inhaled medication will pass through the larynx.

Though stress may play a role in children with PVFD, there is not typically a psychological problem (Brugman & Newman 1993). However, there are reports of PVFD co-occurring with psychiatric disorders such as posttraumatic stress related to sexual abuse, anxiety, and depression (Tajchman & Gitterman 1996, Mullinax & Kuhn 1996).

How the physician makes the diagnosis

Because these attacks occur periodically, it is unlikely that the physician will see the child during one of the symptomatic periods. Physicians most familiar with PVFD and most likely to make the diagnosis include pulmonologists, allergists, and otolaryngologists. The description of the child's symptoms and any pertinent medical history can lead the physician to hypothesize that PVFD is the problem. If the physician happens to see the child during one of the attacks, laboratory results can confirm the diagnosis. In addition, respiratory tests taken during an attack show a change in the shape of the inspiratory loop, called a *blunting of the loop* (asthmatics, on the other hand, have a blunting of the expiratory loop) (Brugman & Newman 1993). Fluoroscopy has also been reported as a method to evaluate glottic function (Nastasi et al. 1997). The gold standard for diagnosing PVFD is visualization of the larynx during an attack. Sometimes physicians will have the child exercise to precipitate an attack, or they administer a medication (methacholine or histamine) to induce PVFD (Brugman & Newman 1993).

Comprehensive Approach to Treatment

Physicians involved in the child's care, any professional providing psychosocial intervention (if needed), and the SLP will work closely to manage the PVFD. Children with PVFD usually respond quickly to the intervention techniques.

The physician's role may include stopping any unnecessary medications the child has been taking (e.g., asthma medications if no asthma is present) and prescribing medication for GERD if necessary. In some instances, anti-anxiety medications may be prescribed, though this is more likely in adolescents than children, and these are often discontinued after the child learns how to control the symptoms.

The SLP's role in PVFD

The SLP has several roles related to children with PVFD. One important role is educating physicians about this disorder which is still often unrecognized. You might consider sending a fact sheet to pediatricians and family practitioners, allergists, pulmonologists, otolaryngologists, and other physicians who treat children. (See Appendix 10A, page 166, for an example fact sheet.) You might offer to talk at a meeting of physicians. Providing education to other adults who might observe these symptoms in children (e.g., teachers who supervise on the playground, coaches) and then refer for medical evaluation would also be invaluable. You may also be the one to ensure compliance with GERD lifestyle changes. (Appendix 4C, page 56, might be helpful.) As an SLP, you are also the professional who provides direct intervention to teach the child how to manage the symptoms.

Treatment usually takes place over a four- to five- week period of time with follow-up as indicated. The sequence described on the next page is a recommended approach. You may have to adjust how much is taught in each session, depending on the age of the child and the child's ability to understand. However, try to make sure that the child leaves the first session with a technique that can be applied during an attack so that she feels a sense of some control over the problem.

Goals for addressing PVFD include:

Long-term goal

Child will be able to engage in all activities without experiencing breathing problems.

Short-term goal

Child will eliminate paradoxical movement of vocal folds occurring during respiration (PVFD).

Treatment Objectives

1. Child will understand physiology of normal inspiration/expiration and the physiology of paradoxical adduction to reduce fear of attacks. (PVFD-1)

2. Child will increase awareness of sensations in throat, pharynx, chest, shoulders, and laryngeal areas. (PVFD-2)

3. Child will utilize pattern of breathing that relaxes muscles of the pharynx: (PVFD-3)
   a. easy exhalation (PVFD-3a)
   b. open throat inhalation (PVFD-3b)
   c. sniff inhalation (PVFD-3c)

4. Child will utilize diaphragmatic breathing paired with relaxed breathing. (PVFD-4)

5. Child will demonstrate reduction of tension in extrinsic laryngeal muscles through a variety of relaxation activities. (PVFD-5)

6. Child will apply these techniques for breathing in a variety of problem situations. (PVFD-6)

Evaluation

PVFD Treatment Objective 1	Child will understand physiology of normal inspiration/expiration and the physiology of paradoxical adduction to reduce fear of attacks.

Mathers-Schmidt (2001) suggests an evaluation comprised of obtaining patient history (PVFD symptoms, pertinent medical history, and social history) and some simple measures of laryngeal and respiratory behaviors:

- Laryngeal valving efficiency and control/respiratory support and control
- Respiratory driving pressure control
- Laryngeal musculoskeletal tension
- Structural/functional integrity of the speech structure

She lists specific rationale for each of these activities, some of which are to demonstrate to the child that she has control of some of these functions. This evaluation is available online at *www.asha.org/journalresources/ajs10020111-fu01.gif*. (Note: If the image is undreadable, expand it by holding the cursor still over the image and waiting for the icon with the arrows to appear. Click on the icon to enlarge the image.)

When a child is seen with a confirmed or strongly suspected diagnosis of PVFD, make sure that the first session includes not only some history-taking, but teaching the techniques the child needs to control the symptoms.

If you are submitting billing to a third party for reimbursement, the most appropriate diagnostic code seems to be 478.75 Laryngeal spasms. If there are related voice problems, consult Chapter 2, page 34. Treatment for PVFD would be coded with the speech therapy code of 92507.

Explaining the problem and your role

The child and her parents may have been told a lot or a little about this problem. The parents may be wondering what an SLP has to do with a breathing problem. If they don't know that SLPs treat voice disorders, it may seem especially foreign to them that you are seeing their child. Explain the nature of the problem and the fact that treatment involves many of the same techniques you use with children who have voice disorders. (If this child has a related voice disorder, it is a secondary concern at this point. Tell the parents you will deal with that after the PVFD attacks are under control). Appendix 10A, page 166, can be used to reinforce what the parents have been told by the physician.

Explain the respiratory system and its relationship to laryngeal movements. Assure the child that although it feels as if she can't get any air in, there is always some air in the lungs. This is important for the child to understand because you will be asking the child to use the air from her lungs to exhale to help release the spasm. Explain how the vocal folds are supposed to move for breathing in and out and show her what her vocal folds are doing during an attack.

Explain that the vocal folds are muscles and that they can get tight and "cramp" just like any other muscle. Ask if the child has ever had a "charley horse" (cramp) in her leg muscle. If so, ask her to remember that if she held her leg in just the right way for just the right amount of time, the cramp went away. Tell her that you will teach her the way to move her laryngeal muscles to make the cramping go away so that the air can come in more easily. If the child has not experienced a leg cramp, ask if she has experienced any pain that felt better when she lay in a certain position or moved in a certain way (e.g., sometimes a stomachache feels better if you curl up).

Prognosis and Typical Progression of Recovery

The child and her parents need to understand that this problem is manageable and should not take long to get under control. If there are no complicating psychosocial issues, the child is typically seen once a week for four to five weeks with follow-up visits scheduled once a month for a few months. Sometimes this follow-up can occur by phone if the child is doing really well. If the child has GERD, the length of treatment may be a little longer while that is being controlled. Most children with PVFD respond immediately to the techniques taught.

Explain to the child that a likely progression will be something like this:

- The child will learn techniques during the first session which will help control the attacks.

- The child may forget to apply the technique until the next attack has started, but then will remember and will try the breathing techniques.

- The child will find that the attack can be stopped fairly easily with the techniques.

- The next time the child feels the tightness starting in her throat, she will immediately use the techniques and will probably stop the attack from happening.

- If the child continues to use the techniques as soon as the tight feeling starts, she will find that the attacks occur less and less frequently.

- If the child practices and applies all the techniques taught and uses other strategies taught (e.g., relaxation, GERD management), it is likely the attacks will occur less and less frequently and may disappear entirely or may happen only on rare occasions.

- The child will be able to handle an attack on those rare occasions.

Recognizing tension

PVFD Treatment Objective 2	Child will increase awareness of sensations in throat, pharynx, chest, shoulders, and laryngeal areas.

To help the child understand the excess tension she may be creating in the structures around the vocal folds, be sure the child understands what you mean by muscle tension. Try a few simple activities like having the child squeeze her fist tightly and then release it. Have her do the same thing with the muscles in her face and then release. Discuss how these same feelings of tension can occur in the larynx, throat, shoulders, etc.

Breathing out and in

PVFD Treatment Objective 3	Child will utilize pattern of breathing that relaxes muscles of the pharynx: a. easy exhalation b. open throat inhalation c. sniff inhalation

Explain to the child that when she feels the tightness in the throat, her first inclination will be to try and breathe in. Tell her that breathing in, especially forcefully, will probably just make the problem worse. Ask if she has ever tried to drink a thick milkshake through a straw and sucked so hard that the sides of the straw collapsed. If not, demonstrate by putting one end of a straw against your finger and sucking on the other end. Explain that if she tries to breathe in, she's actually making the muscles suck in together, just like the straw. Use Appendix 10B, page 167, as a handout as you walk the child through the explanation below.

Tell her that the first thing you want her to do is to breathe out, not breathe in (which is why you laid the groundwork that there is always some air left in the lungs). Acknowledge that this may seem like just the opposite of what she wants to do, but ask her to trust that this will work. Tell her that you want her to breathe out slowly through pursed lips (making a slight blowing sound) or make an "s" sound slowly as she exhales. Remind the child that breathing out is a passive event. That is, as the muscles relax, the air wants to come out. Having the child focus on exhalation should reduce the child's tendency to hold her breath and then struggle to inhale (Martin et al. 1987).

After the child has mastered the slow, relaxed exhalation, tell her you will teach her two ways to breathe in and she can choose the one she likes the best. Many children like the second approach (i.e., sniff) better because it is easier to apply during physical exercise.

Open throat inhalation

This "relaxed-throat breathing" (Brugman & Newman 1993, Martin et al. 1987) focuses the attention away from the larynx and stresses diaphragmatic breathing. With children, you may want to teach the concept of diaphragmatic breathing separately (see Chapter 7, pages 104-105, for more detail). Many children can successfully use open throat inhalation without having to learn about the diaphragm, at least not in the same session. It's more important for the child to feel she is gaining control of her throat muscles. Diaphragmatic breathing can be taught in the next lesson.

Use visual imagery with the child to get her to imagine opening her throat. Have her picture her throat as a wide-open, slick and shiny pipe that air can easily blow through. Then, to have the child understand what you want for tongue position, try teaching this sequence:

- Have the child yawn and ask her to feel what happens in her mouth (the tongue goes to the floor of the mouth, the soft palate elevates). Practice this several times. Ask her to visualize her wide open "pipe" as she is yawning.

- Ask the child to keep her lips (but not her jaw) lightly closed, and "yawn in through your nose." Remind her that her tongue is still going down and her soft palate is going up.

- The child should not take a big, deep breath in. She should breathe in to the count of two. If she tries to take too deep a breath, she may breathe in too fast and trigger closure of the vocal folds.

- If the child is having trouble "feeling" this, try another verbal description. Have her imagine that a balloon is being blown up inside her mouth. In order to make room, her tongue has to move down and the soft palate up.

- When the child has mastered the "open throat/breathing in through the nose," pair it with the slow exhalation through pursed lips or while making the "s" sound.

Sniff inhalation

Another method for encouraging relaxed breathing is to have the child sniff to inhale (Bless 1998). Sniffing almost always utilizes movement of the diaphragm. Explain that the sniffing assures that the vocal folds will open. Sniffing is often preferred over open throat because it can be easily used during physical activity. The pace of the sniffing can be increased as the pace of the activity increases. Try teaching the following sequence:

- Explain that sniffing through the nose will help relax the muscles in the throat, will use the diaphragm for breathing, and will open the vocal folds.

- With her mouth closed, have the child take two quick (and short) sniffs in through the nose.

- Explain that if the child tries to take big sniffs, the pressure might pull the vocal folds back together.

- Have the child place her hand on her abdomen to feel the movement of the abdominal wall (i.e., away from the spine) as she sniffs in.

- When the child has mastered the "sniff/breathing in through the nose," pair it with the slow exhalation through pursed lips or while making the "s" sound.

Always breathe out first

Now that the child has learned one or both of the techniques for breathing in, remind her that when she feels the tightness beginning, she should first breathe out slowly through pursed lips or make the "s" sound as she breathes out. Follow this with one of the methods of breathing in.

Additional work on diaphragmatic breathing

PVFD Treatment Objective 4	Child will utilize diaphragmatic breathing paired with relaxed breathing.

If the child seems to need more work on focusing the breathing away from the throat, utilize detailed information on diaphragmatic breathing found in Chapter 7, pages 104-105. Appendix 7A, page 108, will be a useful handout. This in-depth instruction on diaphragmatic breathing is often left for the second visit.

Exercises to relax the muscles in the shoulders and neck

PVFD Treatment Objective 5	Child will demonstrate reduction of tension in extrinsic laryngeal muscles through a variety of relaxation activities.

Many times, children with PVFD have excess tension in the external muscles of the neck. On the second or third visit, as you continue to reinforce with the child the breathing techniques, you might introduce specific exercises to reduce this tension. Pages 74-75 in Chapter 5 provide background information and Appendix 5C, pages 81-82, is a good handout.

Relaxation exercises

Some children may need more in-depth work on learning to relax in tense situations. They need to learn how to avoid panic attacks and to keep things under control. You may be able to help the child through progressive relaxation exercises and visualization, or you may choose to have the child see another professional (e.g., school counselor, psychologist, licensed clinical social worker) to address this area.

Things to remember during exercise

PVFD Treatment Objective 6	Child will apply these techniques for breathing in a variety of problem situations.

If the child you are working with experiences the attacks during sports activities, you may want to discuss with the child how to use the techniques during physical activity. Appendix 10C, page 168, provides a handout for the child.

Here are some strategies to discuss:

- The child should try to use the breathing techniques throughout the activity and not wait until a problem occurs to start using the open-throat or sniff breathing.
- If the child feels the attack beginning, she should immediately begin the breathing techniques (if not already using them) and consider slowing her pace until she feels she has things under control (e.g., drop back from the action).
- Initially the child may have to come out of the game in order to apply the techniques, but eventually should be able to stay in the game, use the techniques, and keep playing.
- If the child comes out of the game, she must continue the breathing patterns in a "cool down" mode until her breathing has slowed and she no longer feels the tightness in her throat. The coach has to understand this so she doesn't reprimand the child for asking to come out of the game.
- The child might consider slowly walking around on the sidelines as she continues the breathing during this cool-down period.

Applying the skills to real-life situations

Some children seem to be able to apply these skills immediately. Others may need more help with the transition. You may want to help the child practice the skills while moving about. Slowly climbing up and down stairs, walking in the hall, or even going outside for some slow running are good ways to start. Some children may even need you to run with them as they practice the breathing techniques.

Summary

As Mathers-Schmidt (2001) points out, there is much yet to be learned about PVFD, including understanding the triggers and etiologies. We also need to understand why the techniques we use seem to work. PVFD is a serious disorder and children experiencing these attacks understandably are frightened. They need lots of reassurance and encouragement that they can control the problem by learning these techniques and learning to manage other related problems (e.g., GERD, asthma, anxiety).

Vocal Cord Dysfunction Fact Sheet

Paradoxial Vocal Fold Dysfunction (PVFD) is a problem with breathing caused when the vocal folds squeeze together tightly when they should be open and relaxed. This usually happens as the child tries to breathe in, but can happen when the child is breathing out.

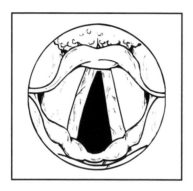 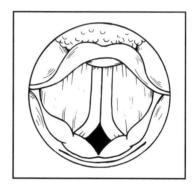

The exact cause of PVFD is not known, but in children these attacks often occur during exercise. They may also be brought on by reflux, panic, and may be related to asthma.

Sometimes children have been diagnosed with severe, uncontrollable asthma when they actually have paradoxical vocal fold dysfunction (PVFD). However, these two problems (PVFD and asthma) can occur together.

Symptoms

- tightness in throat or upper chest
- stridor or noisy breathing
- wheezing
- difficulty swallowing
- shortness of breath
- feels like you can't get air in
- hoarseness

What can be done in therapy?

The speech-language pathologist will use techniques adapted from treatment of voice disorders to teach the child how to gain control of breathing and the opening and closing of the vocal cords. In addition, if the problem is related to stress, some short-term counseling by a psychologist, counselor, or other mental health professional may be helpful for relaxation techniques. The speech-language pathologist will work with the physician, who will treat any related medical problems (e.g., GERD, asthma).

Breathing: Out and In for PVFD

Name _____   Date _____

During a vocal fold dysfunction attack, the front two-thirds of the vocal cords close while you try to breathe in through a small chink in the back one-third. These exercises are designed to help open the vocal cords more completely.

1. Slow easy exhalation

During an attack, the first thing you will be tempted to do is to try to breathe in. You should do just the opposite. You should purse your lips and blow out very slowly. You can also make the "s" sound very slowly as you breathe out.

2. Then use one of these techniques to breathe in.

Open throat inhalation

To practice, first yawn and feel how the soft palate (at the back of the mouth) moves up and the tongue moves down to the floor of the mouth so that the whole mouth feels wide open. Now try yawning with your mouth closed. Your lips should be closed but your teeth should be open and you should try to have the mouth feel wide open like a yawn. Breathe in slowly through your nose. Breathe in to the count of two.

OR

Sniff inhalation

Some children prefer to use the sniff technique for breathing in. This is especially good during physical activities such as sports. Take two quick, short sniffs of air in through the nose. You'll feel your abdomen move out (away from the spine) as you sniff in. Don't take a big sniff.

3. Then slow easy exhalation again.

Breathe out slowly through pursed lips or by making the "s" sound.

4. Continue this sequence until your throat feels relaxed.

Important Tips to Remember During Physical Activity

Name _____   Date _____

Use your techniques all the time.

The best thing to do is use your breathing techniques for all physical activities.

- during practice
- games
- gym class
- running
- climbing steps

If you feel an attack coming on:

As soon as you feel any tightness whatsoever, immediately begin your techniques:

First blow out through your mouth slowly, then take two sniffs in through the nose or open throat breathing to the count of two.

If you feel like your breathing is not relaxing:

Slow your pace a little bit (come to the sidelines, drop back). If you do have to come out of the game or stop your physical activity, be sure to do a cool down. This means that you should slow down (e.g., slower run, quick walk). This is a good time to do shoulder shrugs or shoulder rolls to reduce tension in that area. Remember to keep breathing according to the pattern. Continue until you feel that your breathing is easy and relaxed.

PowerPoint Presentation

You will find this PowerPoint Presentation on the enclosed CD. You can use it to present to a group of children, parents, teachers, and/or coaches. The notes to the right of each slide provide suggestions about activities you can use to expand the presentation and make it more interactive.

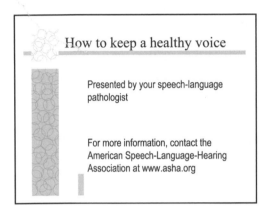

This presentation contains 11 slides. You can present it in as little as 10 minutes, or can extend the length to 20-30 minutes by using the activities. It can be used with preschool children by modifying some of the vocabulary (e.g., referring to the larynx as the *voice box*). It is also appropriate for students up through middle school, as well as for teachers and parents.

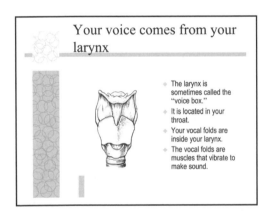

Have students put their hands on their necks and breathe quietly. Point out that they can't feel any buzzing. Then ask them to make a long "z" sound to see if they can feel the vibrations in their necks. Depending on the age of the children, you can give more detailed descriptions of the larynx and use other pictures from the book. For example, you can pass around rubber bands to each child for them to stretch over their fingers like vocal folds. You can talk about how the voice can change in pitch and loudness. You can ask the children to think of cartoon or movie characters who have distinctive sounding voices (e.g., Bugs Bunny).

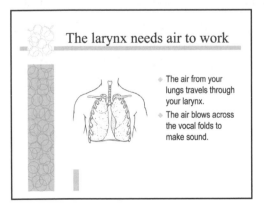

Have a student come to the front of the room and lie down where the other children can see. Use some of the exercises from Chapter 7 (pgs. 102-105) to show the children how the diaphragm works. Have the child who is lying down place a book on his abdomen to demonstrate abdominal wall movement. If there is room, have all the children try this. If not, have the children stand up, take deep breaths, and blow it out slowly while you time how long they can do it.

Pass out balloons to the children. Tell them to use the air from their lungs to fill up the balloons. Then squeeze a balloon at the top to show how air blows across the vocal folds to make sound.

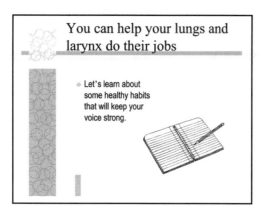

Talk about the different ways that children use their voices: talking to friends at school, at sporting events, on the phone; talking to their family, singing, giving speeches, etc. Solicit input from the students about ways they use their voices. If they provide examples of unhealthy voice uses (e.g., screaming on the playground), use the opportunity to talk about what screaming, loud talking, etc. does to the vocal folds. Talk about things they can do to keep their bodies healthy like getting enough sleep, taking vitamins, and wearing warm clothes when it is cold. Tell them there are also things they should do to keep their voices healthy.

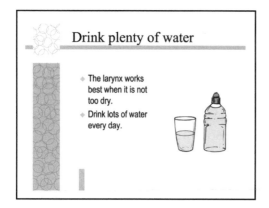

Ask the children to look inside the mouth of the child sitting next to them. Point out how the mouth looks shiny and wet inside. Tell them that the larynx is the same way. It needs to look shiny and wet to work well. A good graphic is to show the children some jelly (or Jell-O) on a plate. Show them how the jelly moves when you shake the plate. Tell them if you let the jelly dry out, it won't be able to wiggle as well.

Ask some of the children how much water they think they drink during a day. Then ask for examples of times they get drinks of water (e.g., after recess). You can also bring in a pitcher and a small glass (e.g., 6 oz.) to show how much water it takes to fill up the pitcher.

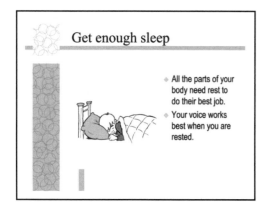

Write some typical bedtimes and wake-up times on the board. Help the children figure out how many hours of sleep are shown (e.g., 8pm-7am). Elicit bedtimes and wake-up times from students to determine how many hours of sleep they get.

Find a picture of a child who looks tired and a child who looks rested. Tell the students that tired child goes to bed at 11:00 and gets up at 6:00 for 7 hours of sleep compared to the rested child who goes to bed at 9:30 and gets up at 6:30 for 9 hours of sleep.

Then ask the children to give examples of days when they haven't had enough sleep and they found it interfered with their performance on something.

170

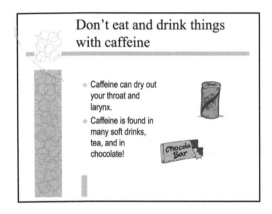

Children may not be familiar with the term *caffeine*, so you may need to explain that it is a chemical that can make things dry out. Explain that caffeine is like a sponge, soaking up all the water they drink. Ask if anyone can tell about a time when their mouth felt really dry. You may need to prompt with questions about coming in after playing on a hot day or when they were sick. Tell them that is what their vocal folds feel like if they have too much caffeine.

You might bring in examples of foods with and without caffeine (e.g., soft drinks, candy) . You could pass out the non-caffeine treat at the end of the presentation.

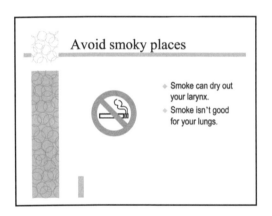

Children are usually familiar with the effects of second-hand smoke. Hopefully, since this presentation is geared for students before adolescence, you won't have any smokers in the audience. You've already talked about how caffeine dries out the vocal mechanism so you can reinforce this message. Talk about why hurting your lungs has an effect on your voice.

You might show students pictures of healthy lungs vs. lungs exposed to cigarette smoke. Such pictures are readily available through the school nurse, American Cancer Society, or the American Lung Association.

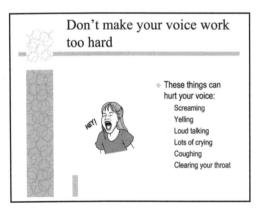

Ask the children for examples of times they have used these abusive behaviors. See if they can think of other examples of things that could hurt their voices. Talk about alternatives to these behaviors. (See Chapter 6, pages 83-100, for more information.)

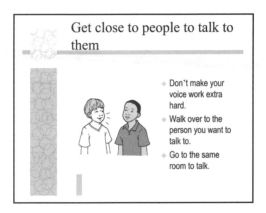

Find out how many children live in homes with more than one floor. Elicit input on how many times the children talk from one floor to another. Ask for examples of other times the children have been far away from someone and tried to talk to them.

Ask for two volunteers and send one to each side of the room. Have them talk to each other. Then ask them what they could do instead of talking across the room. If needed, prompt one of them to walk over close to the other person.

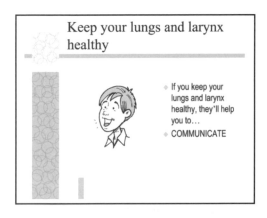

Ask for volunteers in the classroom to be on the Voice Patrol. As a member of the Voice Patrol, they will politely remind others when they hear vocal abuses. Or you might pass out stickers to the whole class and ask them all to join the Voice Patrol.

Resources

The Boone Voice Program for Children
Daniel R. Boone
Pro-Ed, Inc., Austin, TX
1993

Easy Does It for Voice
Catherine Chamberlain and Robin Strode
LinguiSystems, Inc., East Moline, IL
Print by Request
1992

Learning About Voice, Vocal Hygiene Activities for Children:
A Resource Manual
Michael Moran and Elizabeth Zylla-Jones
Thomson Delmar Learning, Clifton Park, NY
1998

The Treatment of Vocal Hoarseness in Children
Julie A. Blonigen
Pro-Ed, Inc., Austin, TX
2000

Visi-Pitch, Nasometer, Sonaspeech
Kay Elemetrics, KayPentax
(800) 289-5297

Vocal Abuse Reduction Program
Thomas S. Johnson
College-Hill Press, San Diego, CA
1985

References

Allen, K. D., Bernstein, B., & Chalt, D. H. (1991). EMG biofeedback treatment of pediatric hyperfunction dysphonia. *Journal of Behavioral Therapy & Experimental Psychiatry, 22*(2), 97-101.

American Speech-Language-Hearing Association. (1998). Roles of otolaryngologists and speech-language pathologists in the performance and interpretation of strobovideolaryngoscopy. *Asha, 40* (Suppl. 18), 32.

American Speech-Language-Hearing Association. (2004). *Preferred practice patterns for the profession of speech-language pathology.* Available at *www.asha.org/members/deskref-journals/deskref/DRVol1.htm*

American Speech-Language-Hearing Association. (2004). Vocal tract visualization and imaging: Position statement. *Asha Supplement 24,* 64.

Andrews, M. (1986). *Voice therapy for children.* New York: Longman.

Andrews, M. L., & Summers, A. C. (2002). *Voice treatment for children & adolescents.* San Diego: Singular/Thomson Learning.

Aronson, A. E. (1990). *Clinical voice disorders: An interdisciplinary approach.* (*3rd ed.*). NY: Thieme Medical Publishers.

Blager, F., Gay, M., & Wood, R. (1988). Voice therapy techniques adapted to treatment of habit cough: a pilot study. *Journal of Communication Disorders, 21,* 393-400.

Bless, D. M., & Swift, E. (1998). *Paradoxical vocal fold dysfunction: When is a paradox not a paradox?* Wisconsin Speech and Hearing Association, University of Wisconsin, Madison: WI.

Bless, E. (1988). Voice disorders in the adult: Assessment. In D. E. Yoder & R. Kent (Eds.), *Decision Making in Speech-Language Pathology* (pp. 136-139). Philadelphia: B. C. Decker.

Bohme, G., & Stuchlik, G. (1995). Voice profiles and standard voice profile of untrained children. *Journal of Voice, 9,* 304-307.

Boone, D. R., McFarlane, S. C., & Von Berg, S. L. (2005). *The voice and voice therapy.* (*7th ed.*). Englewood Cliffs, NJ: Prentice Hall.

Boone, D. R. (1993). *The Boone voice program for children.* Austin, TX: Pro-Ed.

Boone, D. R. (1971). *The voice and voice therapy.* Englewood Cliffs, NJ: Prentice-Hall.

Bouchayer, M., Cornut, G., Witzig, E., Loire, R., Roch, J. B., & Bastian, R.W. (1985). Epidermoid cysts, sucli and mucosal bridges of the true vocal cord: a report of 157 cases. *Laryngoscope, 95,* 1087-1094.

Brodnitz, F. (1971). *Vocal Rehabilitation.* (*4th ed.*). Rochester NY: American Academy of Ophthalmology and Otolaryngology.

References, *continued*

Brugman, S. M., & Newman, K. (1993). Vocal cord dysfunction. *Medical/Scientific Update, 11,* 1-5.

Caraon, P., & O'Toole, C. (1991). Vocal cord dysfunction presenting as asthma. *Irish Medical Journal, 84,* 98-99.

Cheyne, H. A., Nuss, R. C., & Hillman, R. E. (1999). Electroglottography in the pediatric population. *Archives of Otolaryngology-Head & Neck Surgery, 125,* 1105-1108.

Christopher, K. L., Wood, R. P. II, Echkert, R. C., Blager, F. B., Raney, R. A., & Soouhrada, J. F. (1983). Vocal-cord dysfunction presenting as asthma. *The New England Journal of Medicine, 308,* 1556-1570.

Cooper, M. (1973). *Modern trends in voice rehabilitation.* Springfield, IL: Charles C. Thomas.

Deal, R. E., McClain, B., & Sudderth, J. F. (1976). Identification, evaluation therapy, and follow-up for children with vocal nodules in a public school setting. *Journal of Speech and Hearing Disorders, 41,* 390-397.

Eckel, F., & Boone, D. (1981). The s/z ratio as an indication of laryngeal pathology. *Journal of Speech and Hearing Disorders, 46,* 147-149.

Fairbanks, G. (1960). *Voice and articulation drillbook.* New York: Harper & Row.

Glaze, L. E., Bless, D. M., Milenkovic P., & Susser, R. D. (1988). Acoustic characteristics of children's voice. *Journal of Voice, 2,* 312-319.

Glaze, L. E., Bless, D. M., & Susser, R. D. (1990). Acoustic analysis of vowel and loudness differences in children's voice. *Journal of Voice, 4,* 37-44.

Harvey, G. L. (1996). Treatment of voice disorders in medically complex children. *Language, Speech, and Hearing Services in Schools, 27,* 282-291.

Heatley, D. G., & Swift, E. (1996). Paradoxical vocal cord dysfunction in an infant with stridor and gastroesophageal reflux. *International Journal of Pediatric Otorhinolaryngology, 34,* 149-151.

Hillman, R. E., Doyle, P., et al. (1998). *Efficacy of behavioral voice therapy methods for treating women with vocal nodules.* Voice Foundation 27th Annual Symposium: Care of the Professional Voice, Philadelphia, PA.

Hillman, R. E., Gress, C. D., Hargrave, M. S., Walsh, M., & Bunting, G. (1990). Efficacy of speech-language pathology intervention: Voice disorders. *Seminars in Speech and Language, 11*(4), 297-308.

Hillman, R. E., Holmberg, E. B., Perkell, J. S., Walsh, M., & Vaughan, C. (1989). Objective assessment of vocal hyperfunction: An experimental framework and initial results. *Journal of Speech and Hearing Research, 32,* 373-392.

Hillman, R. E., & Verdolini, K. (1999). *Management of hyperfunctional voice disorders: Unifying concepts and strategies.* ASHA videotape.

References, *continued*

Holinger, P. H., & Brown, W. T. (1967). Congenital webs, cysts, laryngoceles and other anomalies of the larynx. *Annals of Otology, Rhinology, and Laryngology, 76,* 744-752.

Holmberg, E. B., Hillman, R. E., & Perkell, J. S. (1989). Glottal airflow and transglottal air pressure measurements for male and female speakers in low, normal and high pitch. *Journal of Voice, 3,* 294-305.

Hull, F. M., Mielke, P. W., Willeford, J. A., & Timmons, R. J. (1976). National Speech & Hearing Survey: Final report (Project 50978). Washington, D. C.: Bureau of Education for the Handicapped, Office of Education, Department of Health, Education, and Welfare.

Iwata, S. (1988). Aerodynamic aspects for phonation in normal and pathologic larynges. In O. Fujimura (Ed.), *Vocal Physiology* (pp. 423-432). NY: Raven Press.

Johnson, T. S. (1985). *Vocal abuse reduction program.* San Diego, CA: College-Hill Press.

Kotby, N. (1995). *The accent method of voice therapy.* San Diego, CA: Singular Publishing Group.

Kotby, M., El-Sady, S., Basiouny, S., Abou-Rass, Y., & Hegazi, M. (1991). Efficacy of the accent method of voice therapy. *Journal of Voice, 5,* 316-320.

Kreiman, J., & Gerratt, B. R. (1998). Validity of rating scale measures of voice quality. *The Journal of the Acoustical Society of America, 104,* 1598-1608.

Kuppersmith, R., Rosen, D. S., & Wiatrak, B. J. (1993). Functional stridor in adolescents. *Journal of Adolescent Health, 14,* 166-171.

Lacy, T. J., & McManis, S. E. (1994). Psychogenic stridor. *General Hospital Psychiatry, 16,* 213-223.

Landwehr, L. P., Wood, R. P. II, Blager, F. B., & Milgrom, H. (1996). Vocal cord dysfunction mimicking exercise-induced bronchospasm in adolescents. *Pediatrics, 98,* 971-974.

Launer, P. G. (1971). Maximum phonation time in children. Unpublished master's thesis, State University of New York at Buffalo.

Lawrence, V. L. (1983). Vocal problems of the professional user of voice. *Seminars in Speech and Language, 4,* 233-244.

Lee, L. (1993). Refocusing laryngeal tone. In J. Stemple (Ed.), *Voice Therapy: Clinical Studies* (pp. 49-53). St. Louis, MO: Mosby Year Book.

Lessac, A. (1973). *The use and training of the human voice,* (3rd ed.). Columbus, OH: McGraw-Hill.

Martin, F. (1988). Tutorial: Drugs and vocal function. *Journal of Voice, 2,* 338-344.

Martin, R. J., Blager, F. B., Gay, M. L., & Wood R. P. II. (1987). Paradoxic vocal cord motion in presumed asthmatics. *Seminars in Respiratory Medicine, 8,* 332-337.

Mathers-Schmidt, B. A. (2001). Paradoxical vocal fold motion: A tutorial on a complex disorder and the speech-language pathologist's role. *Americal Journal of Speech-Language Pathology, 10*, 111-125.

McWilliams, B. J., Bluestone, C. D., & Musgrave, R. H. (1969). Diagnostic implications of vocal cord nodules in children with cleft palate. *Laryngoscope, 79*.

Miller, L. K. (1980). *Principles of everyday behavior analysis*. Monterey, CA: Brooks/Cole Publishing.

Montague, J. C., & Hollien, H. (1973). Perceived vocal quality disorders in Down's Syndrome Children. *Journal of Communication Disorders, 6*, 76-87.

Mullinax, M. C., & Kuhn, W. F. (1996). Benign paradoxical vocal cord adduction presenting as acute stridor. *European Journal of Emergency Medicine, 3*, 102-105.

Mysak, E. D. (1980). *Neurospeech therapy for the cerebral palsied: A neuroevolutional approach (3rd ed.)*. New York: Teachers College Press.

Nastasi, K. J., Howard, D. A., Raby, R. B., Lew, D. B., & Blaiss, M.S. (1997). Airway fluoroscopic diagnosis of vocal cord dysfunction syndrome. *Annals of Allergy, Asthma & Immunology, 78*, 586-588.

Newman, K. B., Mason, U. G. III, & Schmaling, K. B. (1995). Clinical features of vocal cord dysfunction. *American Journal of Respiratory and Critical Care Medicine, 152*, 1382-1386.

Nilson, H. & Schneiderman, C. R. (1983). Classroom program for the prevention of vocal abuse and hoarseness in elementary school children. *Language, Speech, & Hearing in the Schools, 14*(2), 121-127.

Pannbacker, M. (1999). Treatment of vocal nodules: Options and outcomes. *American Journal of Speech-Language Pathology, 8*, 209-217.

Pearl, N. B., & McCall, G. N. (1986). *Laryngeal function during two types of whisper: A fiberoptic study*. Detroit: ASHA Convention.

Perkner, J. J., Fennelly, K. P., Balkissoon, R., Bartelson, B. B., Ruttenber, A. J., Wood, R. P. II, & Newman, L. S. (1998). Irritant-associated vocal cord dysfunction. *Journal of Occupational and Environmental Medicine, 40*, 136-143.

Peterson, K. L., Verdolini-Marston, K., Barkmeier, J. M., & Hoffman, H. T. (1994). Comparison of aerodynamic and electroglottographic parameters in evaluating clinically relevant voicing patterns. *Annals of Otology, Rhonolgy, and Laryngology, 103*, 335-346.

Powell, D. M., Karanfilov, B. I., Beechler, K. B., Treole, K., Trudeau, M. D., & Forrest, L. A. (2000). Paradoxical vocal cord dysfunction in juveniles. *Archives of Otology-Head & Neck Surgery, 126*, 29-34.

Ramig, L., & Verdolini, K. (1998). Treatment efficacy: Voice disorders. *Journal of Speech, Language, and Hearing Research, 41*, 101-116.

Rammage, L. (1996). *Vocalizing with ease: A self-improvement guide.* Vancouver, B. C.: Linda Rammage.

Rammage, L., Morrison, M., & Nichol, H. (2001). *Management of the voice and its disorders (2nd ed.).* Vancouver, CA: Singular/Thomson Learning.

Ringel, R., & Chodzko-Zaijko, W. (1987). Vocal indices of biological age. *Journal of Voice, 1,* 31-37.

Rosin, D. F., Handler, S. D., Potsic, W. P., Wetmore, R. F., & To, L. W. C. (1990). Vocal cord paralysis in children. *Laryngoscope, 100,* 1174-1179.

Roy, N., Bless, D. M., Heisey, D., & Ford, D. N. (1997). Manual circumlaryngeal therapy for functional dysphonia: An evaluation of short and long term treatment outcomes. *Journal of Voice, 11,* 321-331.

Sabol, J. W., Lee, L., & Stemple J. C. (1995). The value of vocal function exercises in the practice regimen of singers. *Journal of Voice, 9,* 27-36.

Sapienza, C. M., Stathopoulous, E. T., & Brown, W. S. (1997). Speech breathing during reading in women with vocal nodules. *Journal of Voice, 11,* 195-201.

Silverman, E. M., & Zimmer, C. H. (1975). Incidence of chronic hoarseness among school-aged children. *Journal of Speech and Hearing Disorders, 40,* 211-215.

Stemple, J., Lee, L., D'Amico, B., & Pickup, B. (1994). Efficacy of vocal function exercises as a method of improving voice production. *Journal of Voice, 8,* 271-278.

Stemple, J., Weiler, E., Whitehead, W., & Komray, R. (1980). Electromyographic biofeedback training with patients exhibiting a hyperfunctional voice disorder. *Laryngoscope, 90,* 471-475.

Stemple, J. C. (2000). Vocal hyperfunction in children: Therapy with limited parental interaction. *Voice therapy: Clinical case studies* (pp. 98-102). San Diego, CA: Singular/Thomson Learning.

Stemple, J. C., Glaze, L., & Klaben, B. G. (2000). *Clinical voice pathology theory and management.* San Diego, CA: Singular/Thomson Learning.

Storms, W. W. (1999). Exercise-induced asthma: Diagnosis and treatment for the recreational or elite athlete. *Medicine & Science in Sports & Exercise, 31* (Suppl. 1), 33-38.

Tajchman, U. W., & Gitterman, B. (1996). Vocal cord dysfunction associated with sexual abuse. *Clinical Pediatrics, 35,* 105-108.

Tan, K. L., Eng, P., & Ong, Y. Y. (1997). Vocal cord dysfunction: Two case reports. *Annals of the Academy of Medicine, Singapore, 26,* 494-494.

Titze, I. R. (1988). The physics of small-amplitude oscillation of the vocal folds. *Journal of the Acoustical Society of America, 83,* 1536-1552.

Van den Berg J. (1958). Myoelastic-aerodynamic theory of voice production. *Journal of Speech and Hearing Research, 1,* 227-244.

van der Merwe, A., (2004). The voice use reduction program. *American Journal of Speech-Language Pathology, 13*, 208-218.

Verdolini, K. (1998). Resonant voice therapy. In K. Verdolini (Ed.), *National Center for Voice and Speech's Guide to Vocology* (pp. 34-35). Iowa City, IA: National Center for Voice and Speech.

Verdolini, K., Titze, I., & Fennell, A. (1994). Dependence of phonatory effort on hydration level. *Journal of Speech and Hearing Research, 37*, 1001-1007.

Verdolini-Marston, K. (1991). *The most common vocal injuries: Nodes and polyps and their causes.* Voice and Speech Trainers Association, Inc., 5(1), 7.

Verdolini-Marston, K., Burke, M. K., Lessac, A., Glaze, L., & Caldwell, E. (1995). Preliminary study of two methods of treatment for laryngeal nodules. *Journal of Voice, 9*, 74-85.

Verdolini-Marston, K., Sandage, M., & Titze, I. R. (1994). Effect of hydration treatments on laryngeal nodules and polyps and related measures. *Journal of Voice, 8*, 30-47.

Warburton, C. J., Niven, R. M., Higgins, B. G., & Pickering, C. A. C. (1996). Functional upper airways obstruction: Two patients with persistent symptoms. *Thorax, 51*, 965-966.

Watkin, K., & Ewanowski, S. (1979). Effects of trimcinolone acetonide on the voice. *Journal of Speech and Hearing Disorders, 22*, 446-455.

Wilson, D. K. (1987). *Voice problems of children.* (3rd ed.). Baltimore, MD: Williams and Wilkins.

Wilson, D. K. (1979). *Voice problems of children.* (2nd ed.). Baltimore, MD: Williams and Wilkins.

Wilson, F. B. (1970). The voice-disordered child: A descriptive approach. *Language, Speech, and Hearing Services in Schools, 4*, 14-22.

Yanagihara, N. (1967). Significance of harmonic changes and noise components in hoarseness. *Journal of Speech and Hearing Research, 10*, 531-41.

Zwitman, D., & Calcaterra, T. (1973). The "silent cough" method for vocal hyperfunction. *Journal of Speech and Hearing Disorders, 38*, 119-125.

23-13-9876